In Search of Turtles Truth in All Vaccination - The Exhaustive Way down Analysis of Vaccine Science Book:

A Comprehensive Exploration of Science, Safety, Myths, and the Global Debate over Immunization

"In Search of Turtles Truth in All Vaccination - The Exhaustive Way down Analysis of Vaccine Science Book"

Library of Congress Cataloging-in-Publication Data

Available upon request.

Disclaimer

The information in this book is intended for educational and informational purposes only. It is not a substitute for professional medical advice, diagnosis, or treatment. Always seek the advice of your physician or other qualified health provider with any questions you may have regarding a medical condition or health goals.

Contact Email: mspublishing2003@gmail.com

Cover Design by Unbreakable Publishers

Printed in USA

Table of Contents

Introduction

Why This Book Matters: Navigating the Vaccine Debate

Vaccination is often touted as one of the most significant achievements in modern medicine. It has saved millions of lives, eradicated diseases like smallpox, and drastically reduced the prevalence of others, such as polio, measles, and diphtheria. Yet, despite its success in preventing disease and improving public health worldwide, vaccination remains a controversial and divisive issue. In recent years, debates about vaccine safety, the ethics of mandatory vaccination, and the role of government in public health have become increasingly heated.

This book exists because, in today's world, navigating the vaccine debate can feel overwhelming. With the rise of misinformation, contradictory opinions, and emotional rhetoric on all sides, how can we, as individuals and as a society, come to clear, rational conclusions about something so fundamental to public health? Whether you're a parent grappling with decisions about your child's vaccination schedule, a health professional seeking a deeper understanding of vaccine safety, or simply someone interested in the science behind the controversy, this book is here to provide clarity and informed insight.

In the age of social media, it's easy to find conflicting stories about vaccines, ranging from claims of harmful side effects to assertions that vaccines are unnecessary or even dangerous. These claims often spread faster than scientific evidence can counter them, leaving many people uncertain or fearful. This book aims to provide a comprehensive, evidence-based approach to these concerns, helping you cut through the noise and understand the science that drives vaccine recommendations.

It is vital that every individual, parent, and healthcare provider has access to reliable, clear, and scientifically sound information about vaccines. Making decisions based on inaccurate or incomplete information can have serious consequences—not only for individuals but for society as a whole. The vaccine debate is not just a personal issue; it is a public health issue, impacting communities and entire nations. Understanding the science behind vaccines—and the myths and misconceptions that surround them—can help ensure that the decisions we make are informed, responsible, and grounded in evidence.

This book is not about promoting one side of the argument over the other, but about presenting a fair and balanced exploration of the facts. By consolidating vast amounts of scientific data, research studies, and expert opinions, this book provides a thorough and thoughtful analysis of vaccine safety, efficacy, and the ethical questions that accompany vaccination policy. You will find more than 1,200 references drawn from peer-reviewed scientific journals, textbooks, and government reports, which offer a foundation of solid evidence that you can rely on.

Ultimately, **this book matters because the vaccine debate is far too important to ignore or misunderstand.** Informed decisions based on credible science lead to better health outcomes for individuals and for society. This book will equip you with the knowledge you need to make those informed decisions—whether you're addressing your own concerns or those of others around you. Together, we can move beyond the myths, mistrust, and misinformation, and find a common ground rooted in truth and scientific integrity.

Understanding the Controversy: A Brief Overview

The debate over vaccination is complex, often characterized by strong emotions, conflicting narratives, and deeply entrenched beliefs. At its core, this controversy centers around two main issues: vaccine safety and the necessity of vaccination. Despite decades of scientific research supporting the effectiveness and safety of vaccines, a vocal group of critics continues to raise concerns, often challenging the very foundation of vaccine policy and public health initiatives.

The Emergence of the Vaccine Debate

The origins of the modern vaccine debate can be traced back to several key events. One of the most pivotal moments came in 1998, when a study published by British doctor Andrew Wakefield in *The Lancet* suggested a link between the MMR (measles, mumps, rubella) vaccine and autism. Although the study was later retracted, and Wakefield lost his medical license due to ethical violations, the damage was done. The idea that vaccines could cause autism gained significant traction among certain groups, fueling widespread fear and mistrust of vaccines.

In the years that followed, other claims emerged, such as allegations that vaccines caused autoimmune disorders, neurological damage, and even sudden infant death syndrome (SIDS). These claims, often amplified by social media and celebrity endorsements, intensified public skepticism and divided communities. The debate was no longer confined to a small group of activists; it had become a mainstream conversation, with serious implications for public health.

The Two Sides of the Vaccine Debate

At the heart of the controversy is the conflict between the medical establishment, which largely supports vaccination, and a growing number of critics, including some doctors, scientists, and parents, who question vaccine safety and necessity.

1. **Pro-Vaccine Position:** The mainstream medical and scientific community firmly supports vaccination, citing overwhelming evidence from decades of research and clinical trials. Vaccines are widely regarded as one of the safest and most effective tools for preventing infectious diseases. In fact, vaccines have been credited with the near-eradication of diseases like smallpox and polio, and have drastically reduced the incidence of other diseases, such as measles

and diphtheria. According to public health organizations like the World Health Organization (WHO) and the Centers for Disease Control and Prevention (CDC), vaccines save millions of lives every year and are considered essential to maintaining herd immunity, which protects vulnerable individuals who cannot be vaccinated.

2. **Anti-Vaccine and Vaccine-Critical Position:** On the other hand, vaccine critics argue that vaccines can cause significant harm, citing instances of adverse reactions, such as allergic reactions, neurological damage, and chronic illnesses, that they believe are linked to vaccination. Some critics assert that vaccine ingredients, such as mercury (in the form of thimerosal), aluminum, and other preservatives, may pose health risks. They argue that vaccine manufacturers are not held accountable for the side effects caused by their products and that clinical trials often fail to adequately demonstrate vaccine safety. Others challenge the necessity of widespread vaccination, questioning why vaccines are recommended for diseases that have become less common due to improved sanitation and public health measures.

The Role of Trust and Misinformation

Central to the controversy is the issue of trust. Many vaccine critics feel that the medical community, pharmaceutical companies, and government health agencies have not been transparent about the potential risks of vaccines. They argue that conflicts of interest, such as financial ties between drug manufacturers and health organizations, skew vaccine research and public health policy in favor of industry interests.

Meanwhile, proponents of vaccination contend that the overwhelming body of evidence supporting vaccine safety comes from a wide range of independent sources and that the benefits of vaccination far outweigh the risks. They argue that the spread of misinformation and conspiracy theories has been fueled by sensational media coverage and the amplification of unverified claims on social media, making it difficult for individuals to distinguish between credible scientific information and baseless fearmongering.

The Impact of the Debate

The vaccine debate has real-world consequences. In recent years, we have seen a resurgence of diseases that were once nearly eradicated, such as measles, due to declining vaccination rates. This is particularly concerning for vulnerable populations, such as infants too young to be vaccinated, the elderly, and those with compromised immune systems, who rely on herd immunity to protect them from preventable diseases. The rise of vaccine-preventable outbreaks highlights the importance of making informed decisions based on evidence and expert guidance.

However, the debate is not just about public health; it also raises important ethical questions. Should vaccination be mandatory? If so, who decides what vaccines are required, and what criteria are used? What role do individual rights and freedoms play in the context of public health measures?

A Path to Understanding

This book aims to provide a balanced, evidence-based exploration of the vaccine debate. By examining the scientific research, medical guidelines, and ethical considerations that underpin the vaccination discussion, we hope to give you the tools you need to critically assess the claims and make informed decisions. Throughout the book, we will address the questions and concerns that many have about vaccine safety, the history of vaccination, and the social and political issues surrounding immunization.

In the end, the goal is not to tell you what to believe but to equip you with the knowledge to understand the complexities of the issue, so you can make decisions based on facts, not fear or misinformation. This book provides you with the scientific references, historical context, and ethical framework needed to navigate the vaccine debate with confidence and clarity.

How This Book Will Help You Find Clarity in the Vaccine Discussion

The vaccine debate is often fraught with confusion, conflicting information, and highly polarized opinions. As the discussion has evolved, it has become increasingly difficult for individuals to sift through the noise and arrive at a clear, evidence-based understanding of the issue. This book is designed to serve as your guide through the complex world of vaccine science, offering clarity and insight in a manner that is both comprehensive and accessible.

A Balanced, Evidence-Based Approach

One of the key ways this book will help you find clarity is by presenting a balanced view of the vaccine debate, grounded in scientific evidence. We do not seek to push an agenda but rather to provide you with the facts, drawn from rigorous scientific research, official publications, and expert opinions. By presenting both the strengths and limitations of the evidence, you will be better equipped to form your own conclusions about vaccine safety, efficacy, and the broader public health implications.

We will explore both the mainstream scientific consensus as well as the concerns raised by vaccine critics, giving you an opportunity to examine the data from all angles. This dual approach will help you see beyond the headlines and sensationalized claims, allowing you to engage with the science in a thoughtful, informed manner.

Unpacking the Complexities of Vaccine Science

Vaccines are a cornerstone of modern medicine, but the science behind them is often misunderstood or oversimplified. Many people are overwhelmed by the technical details or feel disconnected from the research due to a lack of medical background. This book breaks down complex scientific concepts into language that is easy to understand, so you don't need a medical degree to follow along.

We will explore the fundamental principles behind vaccine development, the rigorous processes involved in proving safety and efficacy, and the real-world impact of vaccines on public health. By the end of the book, you will have a solid understanding of how vaccines work, how safety is tested, and why they are such an essential tool for disease prevention.

Clearing Up Common Misconceptions and Myths

A significant portion of the confusion surrounding vaccines stems from widespread myths and misconceptions. Whether it's the claim that vaccines cause autism, that they are a tool for population control, or that they are part of a global conspiracy, there are countless myths that muddy the waters of the vaccine conversation. This book will address these misconceptions head-on, providing you with the facts to debunk myths and false claims.

By dissecting popular myths with evidence-based reasoning, we will help you navigate the overwhelming amount of misinformation in circulation. You will be able to distinguish between credible scientific information and unfounded rumors, empowering you to engage in the discussion with confidence.

Providing Context to the Vaccine Debate

The vaccine debate is not just a scientific discussion but a deeply social, political, and ethical one. In order to fully understand the complexities of the issue, it's crucial to explore the historical and cultural context in which the debate takes place. This book provides you with the necessary background on the history of vaccination, the rise of vaccine skepticism, and the political and social forces that shape public opinion on immunization.

We will also delve into the ethical implications of vaccine mandates, individual rights versus public health, and the role of government agencies and pharmaceutical companies in vaccine policy. By considering these broader issues, you will gain a more nuanced understanding of why the vaccine debate is so contentious and why it matters to society as a whole.

Empowering You with Tools for Decision-Making

Ultimately, this book aims to give you the tools you need to make informed, confident decisions about vaccination. Whether you are a parent trying to navigate the maze of childhood immunizations, a healthcare professional looking for a clearer understanding of vaccine safety, or a concerned citizen wanting to understand the vaccine debate, this book will guide you through the process of gathering evidence, analyzing it critically, and coming to your own conclusions.

Throughout the book, we will provide clear, actionable insights on how to assess the credibility of vaccine research, how to evaluate vaccine safety data, and how to interpret conflicting information. By equipping you with these tools, we aim to empower you to make decisions that align with your values and your understanding of the science, whether that means vaccinating yourself and your family or taking a more cautious approach.

A Comprehensive Resource for Ongoing Learning

The vaccine discussion is constantly evolving, with new research, developments, and public health issues emerging regularly. This book will not only give you the information you need today but will also serve as a lasting resource for future learning. We will provide you with an extensive list of scientific references, key studies, and resources for further reading, so you can continue your exploration of the topic as new evidence comes to light.

By the time you finish reading, you will not only have a clearer understanding of the vaccine debate but will also have the resources and knowledge to stay informed and make decisions based on the best available science.

Summary

In summary, this book is designed to give you clarity in the midst of the vaccine debate by:

- Providing a balanced, evidence-based exploration of vaccine science

- Breaking down complex scientific concepts into clear and digestible explanations

- Debunking myths and misconceptions with factual, peer-reviewed evidence

- Offering historical, social, and ethical context to the vaccine conversation

- Empowering you with the tools to make informed decisions and engage critically with the issue

- Serving as a lasting resource for ongoing education on the topic of vaccines

Whether you are new to the vaccine debate or looking for a deeper understanding, this book will help you navigate the complexities of the discussion and arrive at a well-informed perspective.

Chapter 1: The Science of Vaccination

What Are Vaccines and How Do They Work?

Vaccines are a cornerstone of modern medicine, offering one of the most effective means of preventing infectious diseases. They are designed to protect individuals and communities by stimulating the immune system to recognize and fight specific pathogens, such as bacteria and viruses, without causing the diseases themselves. Understanding how vaccines work involves delving into the fascinating world of immunology, the science of the immune system.

Defining Vaccines

A vaccine is a biological preparation that provides active acquired immunity to a particular infectious disease. It contains components of the pathogen—such as proteins, inactivated virus, or bacterial cells—that trigger an immune response. By introducing these harmless components into the body, vaccines "train" the immune system to recognize and fight the pathogen if encountered again in the future.

There are different types of vaccines, each designed to target specific aspects of a pathogen and to trigger a protective immune response. Vaccines can be made from live but weakened (attenuated) pathogens, inactivated (killed) pathogens, or pieces of the pathogen (such as proteins or genetic material). Regardless of the type, the goal is the same: to prepare the immune system for future encounters with the disease-causing agent.

How Vaccines Work: The Immune System's Role

To understand how vaccines work, it's essential to grasp the basics of how the immune system protects the body from infection. The immune system is a highly specialized network of cells, tissues, and organs that work together to detect and eliminate harmful invaders. It recognizes foreign substances, such as viruses and bacteria, through specialized molecules called antigens.

When the immune system encounters a pathogen, it launches a series of defense mechanisms to fight off the invader. The immune system produces **antibodies**, which are proteins that specifically bind to and neutralize pathogens, preventing them from causing harm. Additionally, the immune system activates **T cells**, which help eliminate infected cells and boost the overall immune response.

Vaccines take advantage of this process by introducing **antigens** from a pathogen into the body in a controlled, harmless way. Here's how this works:

1. **Introducing Antigens**: When a vaccine is administered, it introduces a harmless part of the pathogen into the body. This could be a weakened or inactivated version of the virus, a bacterial toxin, or even just a fragment of the

pathogen (such as a protein). These components are known as **antigens**.

2. **Immune Response**: Upon encountering the antigen, the immune system recognizes it as a foreign substance and mounts a response. This includes the production of **antibodies** that specifically target the introduced antigen. At the same time, the immune system activates **T cells**, which help destroy infected cells.

3. **Memory Formation**: After the immune system has fought off the antigen, it retains a **memory** of the pathogen. Specialized immune cells, known as **memory cells**, store the information about the antigen and remain in the body for long periods, sometimes for a lifetime. This allows the immune system to quickly recognize and respond if it encounters the actual pathogen in the future.

4. **Immunity**: The result of this process is **immunity**—the body's ability to defend itself against future infections by the same pathogen. If the body encounters the real pathogen again, the immune system can launch a rapid and effective response, often preventing illness altogether or minimizing its severity.

Types of Vaccines and Their Mechanisms

Vaccines come in various forms, depending on how they are made and how they trigger the immune response. The main types of vaccines include:

1. **Live Attenuated Vaccines**: These vaccines contain a live but weakened version of the pathogen. Because the pathogen is weakened, it cannot cause disease in healthy individuals but can still stimulate a strong immune response. Examples include the **MMR (measles, mumps, rubella)** vaccine and the **yellow fever** vaccine.

2. **Inactivated (Killed) Vaccines**: These vaccines are made from viruses or bacteria that have been killed or inactivated so that they cannot cause disease. The immune system still recognizes the antigens and produces antibodies, but because the pathogen is dead, it cannot replicate. An example of an inactivated vaccine is the **polio** vaccine.

3. **Subunit, Recombinant, and Conjugate Vaccines**: These vaccines contain pieces of the pathogen—such as proteins, sugars, or toxins—rather than the entire pathogen. By focusing on key parts of the pathogen that trigger the immune system, these vaccines can provide immunity with minimal risk. Examples include the **human papillomavirus (HPV)** vaccine and the **Hib (Haemophilus influenzae type b)** vaccine.

4. **Messenger RNA (mRNA) Vaccines**: A newer type of vaccine, **mRNA vaccines** use genetic material (mRNA) to instruct cells to produce a protein found on the surface of the pathogen. The immune system then recognizes this protein as foreign and responds by producing antibodies.

The **COVID-19 vaccines** from **Pfizer-BioNTech** and **Moderna** are examples of mRNA vaccines.

5. **Toxoid Vaccines**: These vaccines use a toxin produced by a bacteria that has been inactivated to make it harmless. The inactivated toxin triggers an immune response, which prepares the body to neutralize the toxin if it is encountered in the future. Examples include the **diphtheria** and **tetanus** vaccines.

Each type of vaccine has its own strengths and may be chosen based on the nature of the disease, the target population, and the resources available.

Vaccine Administration: How Are Vaccines Given?

Vaccines are most commonly administered through injection, but they can also be given orally or through nasal sprays. The method of administration depends on the type of vaccine and the disease it is meant to prevent.

- **Intramuscular (IM)**: Many vaccines, such as the **flu** and **COVID-19** vaccines, are administered via an injection into the muscle, usually in the upper arm.

- **Subcutaneous (SC)**: Some vaccines, such as the **MMR** vaccine, are injected just under the skin.

- **Oral**: Some vaccines, such as the **oral polio** vaccine, are taken by mouth.

- **Nasal Spray**: The **flu vaccine** is also available as a nasal spray, offering a needle-free alternative for some individuals.

The specific route of administration is chosen based on the vaccine formulation and the type of immunity needed.

Why Vaccines Are Essential: Protecting Individuals and Communities

Vaccines are essential not only for individual protection but also for protecting entire communities. **Herd immunity** occurs when a significant portion of the population is vaccinated, reducing the spread of a disease and protecting individuals who cannot be vaccinated, such as those with compromised immune systems or severe allergies. When enough people are vaccinated, outbreaks are less likely, and the overall public health burden of infectious diseases is reduced.

Vaccination also plays a crucial role in the **eradication** of diseases. For example, the global eradication of **smallpox** and the near-eradication of **polio** were made possible through widespread vaccination campaigns.

Summary

Vaccines are powerful tools that protect individuals and communities from infectious diseases by stimulating the immune system to recognize and fight pathogens. They introduce harmless components of a pathogen (antigens) to trigger an immune response, resulting in immunity and long-term protection. There are several types of vaccines, each designed to work in different ways to offer protection. By understanding how vaccines work, we can appreciate their importance in preventing disease, reducing illness, and saving lives.

The History of Vaccination: From Smallpox to Modern Immunization

The development of vaccination is one of the greatest achievements in the history of medicine, revolutionizing public health and saving millions of lives. Understanding the history of vaccination not only provides context for its current role in disease prevention but also highlights the challenges and triumphs that have shaped the science of immunization over centuries. The story of vaccination stretches from ancient practices to the modern era, with key moments that helped shape its current form.

Early Beginnings: Ancient Practices

The concept of immunization dates back long before the discovery of vaccines. In ancient civilizations, people observed that surviving an infectious disease often resulted in lifelong protection from reinfection. This natural immunity laid the groundwork for early practices designed to protect against diseases.

1. **Variolation**: The earliest recorded use of vaccination-like practices comes from **China** and **India** during the 10th century. In these cultures, a technique known as **variolation** was used to protect people from smallpox. Variolation involved deliberately exposing individuals to material from smallpox sores, typically by inhaling powdered scabs or introducing them into a small cut on the skin. While this method could lead to mild illness, it often resulted in

immunity against the disease without causing death. Variolation spread to the **Middle East** and **Europe** over the centuries, though it was not without risks.

2. **Ancient Egypt**: Some historians argue that ancient Egyptians may have used similar methods to protect against diseases like smallpox, based on depictions of scarring on mummies, suggesting a rudimentary form of inoculation.

Edward Jenner and the Birth of Vaccination

The real breakthrough in vaccination history came in the **18th century**, thanks to **Edward Jenner**, an English physician who discovered the first vaccine. Jenner's work laid the foundation for modern immunization practices.

1. **The Cowpox Experiment (1796)**: Edward Jenner observed that dairymaids who contracted **cowpox**, a mild disease transmitted from cows to humans, seemed immune to smallpox, a deadly disease that had plagued humanity for centuries. Jenner hypothesized that exposure to cowpox might provide protection against smallpox. In 1796, he tested this theory by inoculating an eight-year-old boy with pus from a cowpox lesion. Afterward, he exposed the boy to smallpox, and the boy did not develop the disease. Jenner's experiment proved that cowpox offered immunity to smallpox, marking the birth of the **smallpox vaccine**.

2. **The Term "Vaccination"**: Jenner's success led to the widespread use of cowpox to protect against smallpox, and the term **vaccination** was coined from the Latin word **vacca**, meaning cow. Jenner's discovery revolutionized medicine and marked the beginning of the systematic use of vaccines.

The Fight Against Smallpox: A Global Success

Smallpox was one of the deadliest diseases in human history, but the development of vaccination led to its eventual eradication. In the 19th and 20th centuries, the fight against smallpox became a central focus of public health efforts.

1. **Widespread Adoption of Smallpox Vaccination**: Following Jenner's discovery, vaccination against smallpox became more widely practiced in Europe and North America. The development of more effective and standardized methods for producing the vaccine, such as using calf lymph (cow lymph), helped improve its accessibility and safety.

2. **Global Efforts and Eradication**: In 1967, the **World Health Organization (WHO)** launched a global smallpox eradication campaign. By the early 1970s, smallpox vaccination was widely implemented in many countries, and the disease began to decline sharply. In 1980, the WHO declared **smallpox** eradicated—the first disease to be completely wiped out through vaccination.

Advancements in Vaccination: The 19th and Early 20th Centuries

As the understanding of immunology advanced, so did the development of new vaccines to combat other deadly diseases. These breakthroughs were essential in reducing the global burden of infectious diseases.

1. **Louis Pasteur and Germ Theory**: In the late 19th century, **Louis Pasteur** made groundbreaking contributions to the understanding of germs and their role in disease. Pasteur's work on **germ theory** led to the development of vaccines for diseases like **rabies** and **anthrax**. Pasteur's rabies vaccine, introduced in 1885, was the first vaccine to be developed for a viral infection.

2. **The Development of Diphtheria, Tetanus, and Pertussis Vaccines**: In the early 20th century, **diphtheria**, **tetanus**, and **pertussis** (whooping cough) were major health threats. By the 1920s, vaccines for these diseases were developed, significantly reducing mortality rates and morbidity worldwide. The **DPT vaccine** (Diphtheria, Pertussis, and Tetanus) became a cornerstone of childhood vaccination schedules.

3. **Polio Vaccination**: Perhaps one of the most celebrated achievements in vaccine history was the development of the **polio vaccine**. **Jonas Salk** developed the first **inactivated polio vaccine (IPV)** in the 1950s, followed by **Albert Sabin**, who developed the oral polio vaccine (OPV) in the 1960s. These vaccines were

instrumental in reducing polio cases globally. The continued use of the polio vaccine has led to the near-eradication of polio, with only a few countries still reporting cases.

The Rise of Modern Vaccines: Late 20th Century to Present

The late 20th and early 21st centuries saw the development of a wide range of vaccines targeting new diseases, and the refinement of existing vaccines to make them more effective and accessible.

1. **Vaccine Innovation and New Technologies**: With advancements in biotechnology, new vaccine technologies emerged. The development of **recombinant DNA technology** enabled the creation of vaccines like the **hepatitis B** vaccine, which uses a part of the virus's genetic code to stimulate immunity.

2. **Combination Vaccines**: To simplify vaccination schedules and increase coverage, combination vaccines were developed. These vaccines combine protection against multiple diseases in a single shot. Examples include the **MMR (measles, mumps, rubella)** vaccine and the **DTP (diphtheria, tetanus, pertussis)** vaccine.

3. **Global Vaccination Campaigns**: The WHO and other organizations have worked tirelessly to increase global access to vaccines, focusing on diseases like **measles**, **tuberculosis**, and **hepatitis B**. The introduction of vaccines in low- and middle-income countries has been a crucial

part of global public health efforts, helping to reduce the burden of preventable diseases worldwide.

4. **New Vaccines for Emerging Threats**: As new infectious diseases emerged, such as **HIV/AIDS**, **Ebola**, and more recently, **COVID-19**, the field of vaccinology responded with rapid innovation. The development of **mRNA vaccines** for COVID-19 by companies like **Pfizer-BioNTech** and **Moderna** represents a major leap forward in vaccine technology, with the potential to combat a wide range of diseases more quickly and efficiently.

Conclusion: The Legacy and Future of Vaccination

The history of vaccination is a story of scientific discovery, innovation, and perseverance in the face of disease. From the early days of variolation to the development of modern vaccines, vaccination has played a crucial role in preventing infectious diseases, saving millions of lives, and improving global public health. Today, vaccines continue to be one of the most effective tools in the fight against diseases, with new advancements on the horizon.

As we move forward, the future of vaccination holds promise for addressing emerging infectious diseases, improving vaccine accessibility in underserved regions, and potentially even eradicating more diseases. The legacy of vaccination serves as a reminder of the power of science to protect humanity from the threats posed by infectious diseases, and it highlights the importance of continued investment in vaccine research and development.

The Immune System and How Vaccines Stimulate Immunity

The immune system is a highly complex network of cells, tissues, and organs that work together to defend the body against harmful invaders such as bacteria, viruses, fungi, and parasites. Vaccines take advantage of this system's natural ability to recognize and defend against pathogens, but in a controlled way, to prepare the body for future exposures to these invaders. Understanding how the immune system works and how vaccines stimulate immunity is key to appreciating why vaccination is such a powerful tool in disease prevention.

Overview of the Immune System

The immune system is divided into two main branches:

1. **Innate Immunity**: This is the body's first line of defense, acting quickly and non-specifically to fight off a wide variety of pathogens. It includes physical barriers like skin and mucous membranes, as well as internal defenses such as white blood cells (e.g., neutrophils, macrophages) that attack invaders.

2. **Adaptive Immunity**: This part of the immune system develops more slowly but is highly specific to the pathogens it encounters. It involves specialized cells called **T cells** and **B**

cells that recognize and respond to specific antigens (molecules from pathogens). Once an infection is fought off, the immune system remembers how to respond to that specific pathogen, creating **immunological memory**.

Key Components of the Immune System

Several components of the immune system work in tandem to detect, neutralize, and remember pathogens:

1. **White Blood Cells (Leukocytes)**: These cells play a central role in the immune response. They include:

   o **Macrophages**: Large cells that engulf and digest foreign particles and pathogens.

   o **Dendritic Cells**: These cells capture and process antigens and present them to other immune cells, activating the adaptive immune system.

   o **B Cells**: Produce antibodies, which are proteins that recognize and neutralize pathogens.

   o **T Cells**: Attack infected cells and help regulate the immune response. There are two main types:

      ▪ **Helper T Cells (CD4+ T cells)**: Help activate B cells and cytotoxic T cells.

      ▪ **Cytotoxic T Cells (CD8+ T cells)**: Directly kill infected cells.

2. **Antibodies**: These are proteins produced by B cells that bind to specific antigens on pathogens, marking them for destruction by other immune cells.

3. **Lymphatic System**: This system transports immune cells and fluid throughout the body. The lymph nodes, spleen, and bone marrow are key organs where immune responses are initiated and regulated.

4. **Cytokines**: These signaling molecules coordinate the immune response, helping cells communicate and work together effectively to combat infections.

How Vaccines Work with the Immune System

Vaccines mimic the presence of a pathogen without causing disease, allowing the immune system to "learn" how to defend against it. Here's how vaccines stimulate immunity:

1. **Antigen Introduction**: Vaccines contain antigens that resemble the surface proteins of a virus or bacterium. These antigens are usually harmless because they do not contain the whole pathogen or are weakened forms of it. When a vaccine is administered, the immune system recognizes the antigens as foreign invaders.

2. **Activation of the Immune Response**: The immune system reacts to the foreign antigens by activating the **adaptive immune system**. Specifically:

- o **Dendritic cells** capture the antigens and present them to T cells, activating a targeted immune response.

- o **Helper T cells** then stimulate B cells to produce antibodies specific to the antigens introduced by the vaccine.

- o **Cytotoxic T cells** may also be activated to destroy any infected cells that display the vaccine antigen.

3. **Development of Immunological Memory**: After the immune system has recognized and responded to the vaccine antigens, it retains a memory of how to recognize these antigens in the future. **Memory B cells** and **memory T cells** are created, which "remember" the pathogen. If the body is later exposed to the actual pathogen, these memory cells will quickly recognize and respond to it, preventing illness or reducing its severity.

4. **Long-Term Immunity**: Over time, the immune system retains the ability to quickly produce antibodies and deploy T cells against the pathogen. The duration of immunity varies depending on the vaccine and the pathogen, but in many cases, it provides long-lasting protection.

Types of Vaccines and Their Mechanisms

Different types of vaccines stimulate immunity in various ways, depending on the kind of antigen they contain and the immune response they are designed to elicit. These include:

1. **Inactivated or Killed Vaccines**: These vaccines contain viruses or bacteria that have been killed or inactivated so they cannot cause disease. Examples include the **polio vaccine** (IPV) and **hepatitis A vaccine**. They stimulate the immune system to produce antibodies and memory cells.

2. **Live Attenuated Vaccines**: These vaccines contain weakened forms of the virus or bacterium. While they can replicate and stimulate an immune response, they do not cause illness in healthy individuals. Examples include the **measles, mumps, rubella (MMR)** vaccine and the **yellow fever vaccine**.

3. **Subunit, Recombinant, and Conjugate Vaccines**: These vaccines use specific pieces of the pathogen (like proteins or sugars) rather than the whole organism. These components are carefully chosen to trigger the immune system's response without causing disease. Examples include the **human papillomavirus (HPV)** vaccine and the **Hib vaccine** (for Haemophilus influenzae type b).

4. **Messenger RNA (mRNA) Vaccines**: A newer type of vaccine, mRNA vaccines contain messenger RNA that instructs cells to produce a protein similar to the one found on the surface of the virus (e.g., the spike protein in **SARS-CoV-2**, the virus responsible for COVID-19). The immune system recognizes this protein as

foreign and mounts an immune response. mRNA vaccines do not contain live virus and cannot alter the body's DNA. Examples include the **Pfizer-BioNTech** and **Moderna COVID-19 vaccines**.

5. **Toxoid Vaccines**: These vaccines use inactivated toxins produced by bacteria. The immune system learns to recognize and neutralize the toxin. Examples include the **tetanus** and **diphtheria** vaccines.

Why Vaccines Are Effective in Preventing Disease

Vaccines are effective because they equip the immune system with the knowledge it needs to defend against pathogens. By stimulating the immune system to recognize and respond to an infectious agent, vaccines essentially "train" the body's defenses without causing harm. The **herd immunity** effect—when a large proportion of a population becomes immune to a disease—helps protect those who cannot be vaccinated, such as individuals with certain health conditions or those who are too young.

Vaccination has led to the **eradication of smallpox** and a dramatic reduction in diseases like **measles, polio**, and **whooping cough**. By preventing the spread of infectious diseases, vaccines not only protect individuals but also contribute to the overall health and safety of communities.

Challenges in Vaccination and Immunity

While vaccines are highly effective, no vaccine is 100% perfect. Some individuals may have weakened immune systems due to medical conditions or treatments, making them less responsive to vaccines. Additionally, some diseases can mutate over time, which can impact the effectiveness of vaccines. However, ongoing research and updates to vaccine formulas help to address these challenges and ensure that vaccines remain a crucial tool in disease prevention.

Conclusion

The immune system's ability to recognize and destroy harmful invaders is one of the body's most powerful defenses, and vaccines enhance this ability by preparing the immune system in advance. Through various types of vaccines—whether inactivated, live-attenuated, subunit, or mRNA—immunization teaches the immune system to identify and fight off pathogens without causing harm. This preventive measure has revolutionized public health, saving millions of lives, and remains one of the most effective ways to protect individuals and communities from infectious diseases.

Scientific Foundations of Vaccine Safety and Effectiveness

Vaccines are one of the most significant advancements in public health, preventing countless diseases and saving millions of lives globally. The science behind vaccine development, safety, and effectiveness is extensive, grounded in rigorous research and testing, and continuously evolving to ensure that vaccines provide safe and lasting protection. Understanding these scientific foundations is crucial for appreciating why vaccines are both safe and effective for the vast majority of people.

How Vaccine Safety is Assessed

Ensuring vaccine safety is one of the highest priorities in vaccine development. Before any vaccine is approved for public use, it undergoes several stages of clinical trials designed to rigorously evaluate its safety profile. This process involves:

1. **Preclinical Testing**:

    o   Before testing a vaccine on humans, researchers conduct preclinical studies, usually using animal models, to assess the potential risks and side effects. These studies help scientists understand the immune response generated by the vaccine and whether it causes any harmful effects.

2. **Clinical Trials (Phases 1-3)**:

    o   **Phase 1**: The first phase of clinical trials involves a small group of healthy volunteers, usually under 100 people. It focuses on the vaccine's safety, appropriate dosage, and its ability to trigger an immune response.

    o   **Phase 2**: This phase expands the trial to a larger group (hundreds of individuals). The goal is to further assess safety, optimal dosage, and to begin evaluating the vaccine's ability to protect against the disease in a more diverse population.

- **Phase 3**: In this phase, the vaccine is tested on thousands of participants. The focus is on collecting data about its safety, effectiveness, and potential side effects in a larger, more diverse group of people. This phase is crucial in determining whether the vaccine offers significant protection against the targeted disease and how it compares to a placebo or other treatments.

3. **Post-Marketing Surveillance (Phase 4)**:

- After approval, vaccines are continually monitored for any adverse effects in the general population. This phase is crucial because it allows scientists to detect very rare side effects that might not have appeared during clinical trials, which involve a more limited population.

- **Vaccine Adverse Event Reporting System (VAERS)** in the U.S. and other similar systems worldwide play an important role in tracking vaccine safety in real-world conditions. These systems collect reports of any side effects following vaccination, allowing health authorities to investigate and respond promptly to potential safety concerns.

4. **Ongoing Research and Data Collection**:

o Vaccine safety is continually studied, and new findings are incorporated into vaccine recommendations. For instance, new data on the long-term effectiveness of vaccines may lead to updated guidelines on vaccine schedules, booster shots, or other interventions.

Effectiveness of Vaccines: The Science Behind Immunization

Vaccine effectiveness refers to how well a vaccine prevents disease in a real-world setting. It is measured by studying the rate of disease in vaccinated individuals compared to those who are unvaccinated. Several factors contribute to the effectiveness of a vaccine, including how the immune system responds, the nature of the pathogen, and how widely the vaccine is administered. Key factors influencing vaccine effectiveness include:

1. **Immunological Response**:

   o **Humoral Immunity (Antibody Production)**: Many vaccines stimulate B cells to produce antibodies that specifically target and neutralize pathogens. These antibodies "remember" the pathogen and can rapidly respond if the body encounters it again.

   o **Cell-Mediated Immunity**: Some vaccines also activate T cells, which are responsible for identifying and destroying infected cells. This type of immune response is essential for clearing infections that do not involve antibodies, such as viruses that invade cells directly.

- o **Immunological Memory**: One of the key features of vaccines is their ability to induce long-lasting immunity. After vaccination, the immune system creates **memory cells** (memory B cells and memory T cells) that "remember" the specific pathogens. These cells can rapidly respond to the pathogen if encountered again, providing immunity against future infections.

2. **Vaccine Efficacy in Clinical Trials**:

- o Vaccine efficacy is typically measured during clinical trials. For instance, if a vaccine prevents 90% of infections in a trial, it is said to have an efficacy of 90%. This number is derived from comparing the number of infections in vaccinated participants to those in unvaccinated participants over the course of the study.

3. **Herd Immunity**:

- o When a large portion of a population becomes immune to a disease (either through vaccination or previous infection), the spread of the disease slows down because there are fewer people for the pathogen to infect. This concept, known as **herd immunity**, is critical for protecting individuals who cannot be vaccinated, such as those with compromised immune systems or infants who are too young to receive certain vaccines. Achieving herd immunity requires high vaccination coverage rates.

4. **Vaccine Effectiveness Over Time**:

   o Some vaccines may lose effectiveness over time, which is why booster shots may be recommended. The protection from vaccines like **diphtheria, tetanus**, and **whooping cough** decreases over time, and booster doses help "remind" the immune system to produce a strong defense.

   o For diseases caused by viruses that mutate frequently, such as **influenza** or **COVID-19**, vaccines may need to be updated periodically to protect against the latest strains of the virus.

5. **Real-World Effectiveness**:

   o The real-world effectiveness of vaccines can vary based on several factors, including the population being vaccinated, the timing of vaccine administration, and the overall health of individuals. However, even in imperfect conditions, vaccines have consistently shown to reduce the incidence and severity of disease.

- COVID-19 vaccines, for example, were shown in clinical trials to be highly effective in preventing severe illness, hospitalization, and death. In real-world data, while the vaccines may not always prevent mild illness, they significantly reduce the risk of severe outcomes.

Factors Influencing Vaccine Safety and Effectiveness

While vaccines are generally safe and effective, there are certain factors that can affect their safety and efficacy in individuals:

1. **Age**:
   - Children and the elderly may have different immune responses to vaccines. For example, infants may need to receive several doses of vaccines in a series to build up immunity, while older adults may require higher vaccine dosages or adjuvants to enhance their immune response.

2. **Underlying Health Conditions**:
   - People with certain medical conditions, such as autoimmune diseases, cancer, or immune deficiencies, may have altered immune responses to vaccines. In some cases, individuals with weakened immune systems may not respond as well to vaccination or may need special considerations, such as a different vaccine type or additional doses.

3. **Vaccine Adjuvants**:

    o   Some vaccines contain **adjuvants**, which are substances that enhance the body's immune response to the antigen in the vaccine. While adjuvants improve vaccine effectiveness, some individuals may experience mild side effects related to these components.

4. **Genetic Factors**:

    o   Genetic factors can also influence an individual's response to vaccines. Some people may have a naturally stronger or weaker immune response to certain antigens, which could affect how well they are protected by a vaccine.

The Science of Vaccine Monitoring and Improvements

Vaccine safety and effectiveness are not static; they are subjects of ongoing research and monitoring. As new diseases emerge, or as viruses evolve, vaccines are continuously assessed and updated to ensure optimal protection. The scientific community remains vigilant, continuously working to improve vaccines' safety profiles, adapt to new pathogens, and enhance their effectiveness.

Through **global vaccine surveillance systems**, ongoing studies, and advances in immunology, scientists and health authorities ensure that vaccines continue to be one of the most effective tools in preventing disease and protecting public health.

Whether it's improving existing vaccines, creating new ones, or responding to emerging health threats, vaccine science is always evolving to meet the challenges of a changing world.

Conclusion

The scientific foundations of vaccine safety and effectiveness are built on decades of rigorous research and real-world evidence. Vaccines are designed to safely stimulate the immune system to recognize and defend against pathogens, and their effectiveness is continually assessed through clinical trials, real-world data, and ongoing surveillance. By understanding how vaccines work, how they are tested, and how they contribute to public health, individuals can better appreciate the value of vaccination in preventing disease, protecting vulnerable populations, and maintaining global health.

Chapter 2: The Process of Vaccine Development

The Stages of Vaccine Development: From Lab to Market

The journey of a vaccine from conception to distribution is a lengthy and intricate process, involving a series of critical stages that ensure safety, efficacy, and public health benefits. This chapter will walk you through each stage of vaccine development, shedding light on the exhaustive testing and regulatory oversight that accompanies the creation of a vaccine. From the initial laboratory research to large-scale production and global distribution, we will explore the key milestones in bringing a vaccine to market.

1. Early Research and Discovery

The vaccine development process begins with scientific research aimed at understanding the disease and its causative agent, such as a virus or bacteria. The goal is to identify the specific part of the pathogen (antigen) that can provoke a protective immune response without causing the disease.

- **Pathogen Identification**: Researchers first identify the pathogen responsible for the disease. This involves isolating and studying the microorganism to understand its biology and how it infects humans.

- **Understanding the Immune System's Response**: Scientists examine how the immune system reacts to this pathogen, focusing on the immune cells and molecules that can neutralize or destroy the pathogen. This information helps pinpoint which part of the pathogen should be targeted in the vaccine.

2. Vaccine Design and Preclinical Testing

Once the pathogen has been studied, scientists work on designing the vaccine. There are different approaches for creating vaccines, such as using inactivated viruses, weakened live viruses, protein subunits, or even genetic material like RNA. During the design phase, a prototype vaccine is created, and laboratory tests are conducted.

- **Vaccine Platforms**: Depending on the pathogen, a variety of vaccine types may be designed:
  - **Live Attenuated Vaccines**: Weakened forms of the virus or bacteria.
  - **Inactivated Vaccines**: Killed versions of the pathogen.
  - **Subunit, Recombinant, or Conjugate Vaccines**: Parts of the pathogen or its antigens.
  - **mRNA Vaccines**: Genetic material that instructs cells to produce the target antigen.
  - **Viral Vector Vaccines**: Use a harmless virus to deliver genetic material from the pathogen.

- **Preclinical Testing**: Before testing on humans, vaccines undergo preclinical testing using animal models. This helps scientists determine the vaccine's safety and potential to induce an immune response. These tests also provide important data on optimal dosage, route of administration, and possible side effects.

3. Clinical Trials: Phases 1, 2, and 3

If preclinical testing is successful, the vaccine enters human clinical trials, which occur in three phases. Clinical trials are designed to evaluate the safety, efficacy, and proper dosage of the vaccine, with each phase involving more participants.

- **Phase 1: Safety and Immune Response**
  - Phase 1 trials focus on a small group of healthy volunteers (usually fewer than 100). The primary goal is to determine the vaccine's safety and assess whether it provokes an immune response. Researchers monitor for side effects, both short-term and long-term, and evaluate the correct dosage for further trials.

- **Phase 2: Expanding Safety and Efficacy Testing**
  - Phase 2 trials involve hundreds of participants, including individuals from different demographic groups (such as children, elderly, or people with underlying conditions). The focus of this phase is on evaluating the vaccine's

ability to produce a strong immune response and testing it in a broader population. It also aims to refine dosing schedules and investigate possible side effects in a larger group.

- **Phase 3: Efficacy and Large-Scale Safety**

  o Phase 3 trials are the largest and most pivotal. Thousands of participants are tested, including those from diverse populations. This phase measures the vaccine's ability to protect against the disease in the general population. Researchers compare the number of disease cases in vaccinated participants versus those who receive a placebo. The focus is on confirming the vaccine's safety, its effectiveness in preventing the disease, and identifying any rare side effects.

4. Regulatory Review and Approval

After successful completion of Phase 3, the vaccine's data is submitted to regulatory authorities for review. Agencies like the **U.S. Food and Drug Administration (FDA)**, the **European Medicines Agency (EMA)**, and the **World Health Organization (WHO)** scrutinize all the clinical trial data, including safety and efficacy results, as well as the manufacturing process.

- **Data Evaluation**: Regulatory bodies assess whether the vaccine meets rigorous safety standards and if the benefits outweigh any potential risks. If the vaccine is found to be safe and effective, it is granted approval for public use. Some vaccines may be approved for emergency use if they meet specific criteria, particularly during global health crises like pandemics.

- **Approval for Use**: Once approved, the vaccine can be distributed and made available to the public. However, approval does not end the monitoring process. Post-market surveillance continues to ensure ongoing safety.

5. Manufacturing and Production

Once a vaccine is approved, the production phase begins. Scaling up from laboratory quantities to millions (or even billions) of doses is a complex task that involves establishing large-scale manufacturing facilities and implementing strict quality control measures. The following steps are essential in this phase:

- **Manufacturing Scale-Up**: Vaccine production is scaled up, and it must adhere to Good Manufacturing Practices (GMP) to ensure consistency, safety, and quality across every batch. This phase can take several months and may require the expansion of manufacturing capabilities to meet global demand.

- **Quality Control**: Vaccines are subjected to a variety of tests to ensure they meet quality standards. These tests check for contamination, potency, and stability.

- **Cold Chain Requirements**: Some vaccines, particularly those like mRNA vaccines, need to be stored and transported at very low temperatures to remain stable. Establishing an efficient cold chain network is critical to preserving vaccine quality during transportation.

6. Distribution and Deployment

Once vaccines are produced and packaged, they are distributed to healthcare providers, government agencies, and international organizations. The distribution phase involves logistical planning to ensure vaccines reach their destinations, particularly in rural or hard-to-reach areas.

- **Global Distribution Efforts**: Organizations like **COVAX** work to ensure that vaccines are distributed equitably, especially in low- and middle-income countries. Global health initiatives aim to reduce disparities in vaccine access to ensure that all populations can benefit from vaccination programs.

- **Vaccine Delivery**: Vaccines are delivered to local clinics, hospitals, and vaccination centers, where healthcare professionals administer them. Governments and healthcare systems must work together to ensure that vaccinations are provided quickly and efficiently, particularly in the case of pandemic outbreaks.

7. Post-Market Surveillance

Even after a vaccine is authorized and distributed, it is still closely monitored for any adverse effects or long-term safety concerns. Post-market surveillance helps to identify rare side effects that may not have been detected in clinical trials, especially those that occur only after the vaccine has been administered to large numbers of people.

- **Vaccine Adverse Event Reporting System (VAERS)**: In many countries, including the U.S., reporting systems like VAERS allow healthcare providers and the public to report any potential side effects after vaccination. This data is then reviewed to identify patterns and respond quickly to potential safety concerns.

- **Ongoing Research**: Manufacturers continue to collect data on the vaccine's long-term effectiveness, and health authorities may recommend booster shots or modified schedules based on emerging data.

8. Continuous Improvement and Adaptation

As new variants of a disease-causing pathogen emerge or new health concerns arise, vaccines may need to be updated or adapted. For example, flu vaccines are updated each year to match the circulating strains of the influenza virus. Similarly, COVID-19 vaccines have been updated to address new variants of the SARS-CoV-2 virus.

- **Booster Shots**: In some cases, vaccine manufacturers and health authorities recommend booster doses to reinforce immunity and protect against new strains of a virus.

- **Vaccine Research and Innovation**: Scientists continue to explore new vaccine technologies and platforms, aiming to create more effective, accessible, and globally distributable vaccines.

Conclusion

The stages of vaccine development, from initial discovery through clinical trials to mass production and post-market surveillance, are critical in ensuring that a vaccine is safe, effective, and accessible to the global population. While the process may seem lengthy and complex, it is a necessary part of protecting public health and preventing the spread of infectious diseases. Understanding the science and the extensive steps involved in vaccine development highlights the efforts of scientists, public health officials, and healthcare professionals in safeguarding global health.

Testing for Safety: How Vaccine Trials Are Conducted

Vaccine trials are essential for ensuring that vaccines are both safe and effective before they are distributed to the general public. These trials are conducted in several stages, each of which plays a critical role in confirming the safety and immunogenicity of a vaccine. In this section, we will explore how safety is rigorously tested at each stage of vaccine trials, the different methods used to monitor and evaluate safety, and the ethical considerations that guide these trials.

1. The Ethical Foundations of Vaccine Trials

Before any vaccine trial begins, ethical guidelines ensure that participant safety is prioritized. These guidelines are governed by international standards such as the **Declaration of Helsinki** and are enforced by ethical review boards (IRBs) that oversee clinical research.

- **Informed Consent**: All participants must be fully informed of the potential risks and benefits of the trial. They must voluntarily agree to participate without any coercion, understanding the nature of the vaccine, the testing process, and their right to withdraw at any time.

- **Balancing Risk and Benefit**: Researchers must carefully assess the balance between the potential benefits of the vaccine (protection against disease) and the risks (side effects or adverse events). This evaluation helps to ensure that the benefits outweigh the potential harms, particularly in vulnerable populations.

2. Phase 1: Initial Safety Testing in a Small Group

Phase 1 clinical trials are the first stage of testing a new vaccine in humans. The goal of Phase 1 is primarily to assess the safety of the vaccine and determine whether it induces a sufficient immune response. In this phase:

- **Participants**: A small group of healthy volunteers, typically fewer than 100 individuals, is selected. These participants are usually adults, and some trials may include diverse demographic groups.

- **Safety Monitoring**: The focus is on detecting any immediate or short-term side effects or adverse reactions. Volunteers are monitored closely after vaccination for reactions such as fever, redness, swelling, or pain at the injection site.

- **Dose Determination**: Researchers determine the optimal dose by testing multiple doses of the vaccine. This phase helps identify the lowest effective dose that provides an adequate immune response without significant side effects.

- **Immune Response Evaluation**: Blood samples are taken to assess the immune system's response to the vaccine. Researchers check whether the vaccine has induced the production of antibodies or stimulated other immune cells that can fight the pathogen in question.

3. Phase 2: Expanded Safety Testing in a Larger Group

Phase 2 trials involve hundreds of participants and are designed to expand the safety testing of the vaccine while further assessing its ability to trigger an immune response. Key aspects of Phase 2 trials include:

- **Participants**: Phase 2 trials usually involve several hundred participants from various demographic groups (age, sex, underlying health conditions). This phase is more inclusive than Phase 1, offering better insight into how the vaccine performs in a broader population.

- **Monitoring for Adverse Events**: Researchers continue to closely monitor participants for any adverse reactions, including those that may be less common or delayed. Participants are observed for any serious side effects such as allergic reactions, neurological symptoms, or any long-term health concerns.

- **Longer Follow-Up**: Phase 2 trials generally last for a few months to identify any delayed or long-term side effects. Participants are asked to report any health issues they experience, and researchers follow up regularly to track their health outcomes.

- **Evaluating Immunogenicity**: This phase also assesses the immune response in more detail. Researchers study not only the quantity of antibodies produced but also the quality of the immune response, such as whether the vaccine can trigger the production of specific antibodies that target different parts of the pathogen.

4. Phase 3: Large-Scale Efficacy and Safety Testing

Phase 3 trials are the largest and most critical stage in the clinical trial process. They are conducted with thousands of participants and focus on confirming the vaccine's safety and efficacy. This phase provides the most comprehensive data on a vaccine's performance.

- **Participants**: Phase 3 trials involve thousands of participants, often across multiple regions and countries. Participants are selected to be representative of the general population, including individuals with a range of health conditions, ages, and other risk factors.

- **Randomized Control Trials (RCTs)**: In most Phase 3 trials, participants are randomly assigned to either the vaccine group or a placebo group (a group that receives a non-active substance). This helps eliminate bias and provides a clearer comparison of outcomes between those who received the vaccine and those who did not.

- **Adverse Event Monitoring**: Researchers closely monitor all participants for any adverse effects. Serious adverse events (SAEs), such as life-threatening allergic reactions or unexpected health problems, are carefully documented and investigated. These events are compared between the vaccine group and the placebo group to determine if there is an association with the vaccine.

- **Efficacy Testing**: The primary goal of Phase 3 trials is to determine whether the vaccine is effective at preventing the disease in the general population. This is done by measuring how many people in the vaccine group contract the disease compared to the placebo group. Efficacy is often reported as a percentage, indicating how much less likely vaccinated individuals are to contract the disease compared to unvaccinated individuals.

- **Safety Review Committees**: Independent safety monitoring boards, often referred to as Data Safety Monitoring Boards (DSMBs), oversee Phase 3 trials to ensure that any unexpected side effects are detected and properly evaluated. These committees can halt a trial if a serious safety issue arises.

5. Emergency Use Authorization (EUA) and Post-Market Surveillance

In some cases, especially during global health emergencies, a vaccine may be granted **Emergency Use Authorization (EUA)** before completing all Phase 3 trial steps. This allows the vaccine to be distributed rapidly, often to at-risk populations.

- **Emergency Use**: Under EUA, regulatory agencies like the FDA or EMA may approve the vaccine based on the available data from earlier phases, provided the benefits outweigh the risks. These vaccines are still closely monitored and additional data may be collected post-marketing.

- **Post-Market Surveillance (Phase 4)**: After a vaccine is approved and distributed to the public, ongoing surveillance continues. This phase includes the monitoring of long-term safety and efficacy in the general population. Vaccine recipients are encouraged to report adverse events, and regulatory agencies review this data to ensure the vaccine remains safe.

6. Risk Communication and Informed Decision-Making

Throughout the vaccine trial process, clear and transparent communication about potential risks and benefits is vital. Regulatory bodies, public health officials, and researchers must ensure that the public is informed about:

- **Common Side Effects**: The most common side effects of vaccination are usually mild and temporary, such as soreness at the injection site, fever, or fatigue.

- **Rare Adverse Events**: Any rare or serious side effects, such as anaphylaxis (severe allergic reaction), must be reported promptly. Public health officials provide guidance on how to manage these risks.

- **Benefit-Risk Assessment**: Regulatory bodies weigh the benefits of vaccination (prevention of disease, public health protection) against the risks (potential side effects) to make informed decisions about vaccine approval.

Conclusion

Vaccine safety is a top priority throughout the development process, and vaccine trials are conducted with rigorous oversight to ensure that vaccines are both effective and safe for widespread use. The various phases of clinical trials—starting with small groups and progressing to large, diverse populations—provide comprehensive data on the vaccine's safety, immune response, and potential risks. Even after approval, vaccines undergo continuous monitoring to detect any long-term or rare side effects. This thorough testing process builds public confidence in the vaccines that help protect individuals and communities from infectious diseases.

Regulatory Oversight: The Role of Health Authorities in Vaccine Approval

The approval and regulation of vaccines are critical to ensuring that they are safe, effective, and suitable for public use. Health authorities and regulatory agencies play an essential role in overseeing the entire vaccine development process, from initial research to post-market surveillance. This section explores the role of these regulatory bodies in approving vaccines and their responsibilities in maintaining public health safety.

1. Key Regulatory Bodies Involved in Vaccine Approval

Several major health authorities around the world are responsible for overseeing vaccine safety, efficacy, and quality. These regulatory agencies ensure that vaccines meet rigorous standards before being authorized for public use.

- **The U.S. Food and Drug Administration (FDA)**: In the United States, the FDA is the primary regulatory agency for vaccine approval. It evaluates the safety and efficacy of vaccines through its **Center for Biologics Evaluation and Research (CBER)**, which reviews clinical trial data and ensures that vaccines meet specific manufacturing and labeling standards.

- **The European Medicines Agency (EMA)**: In the European Union, the EMA evaluates vaccines through its **Committee for Medicinal Products for Human Use (CHMP)**. The agency is responsible for providing scientific recommendations for vaccine approval and monitoring their safety once they are in use.

- **The World Health Organization (WHO)**: The WHO sets international standards for vaccine safety and efficacy and provides guidance on vaccine development, evaluation, and use. It also coordinates efforts to ensure that vaccines are accessible in low- and middle-income countries.

- **Other National Health Authorities**: Many countries have their own regulatory agencies, such as **Health Canada**, **Medicines and Healthcare products Regulatory Agency (MHRA)** in the UK, and **TGA (Therapeutic Goods Administration)** in Australia. These agencies follow similar procedures to the FDA and EMA, evaluating clinical trial data and post-market safety monitoring.

2. Pre-Approval Process: Review and Evaluation of Vaccine Data

Before a vaccine is approved for public use, health authorities conduct a thorough review of the vaccine's clinical trial data. This process involves several key steps:

- **Data Submission**: Vaccine developers submit all data from preclinical studies and clinical trials to the regulatory agency. This includes detailed reports on the safety, efficacy, and quality of the vaccine, as well as information on how it was manufactured.

- **Scientific Review**: Regulatory agencies assemble teams of scientists, medical experts, and statisticians to review the vaccine data. They assess the vaccine's ability to stimulate immunity, its safety profile, and whether it provides protection against the targeted disease.

- **Consultation with Advisory Committees**: In many cases, health authorities convene advisory committees of independent experts to review the data and make recommendations on whether the vaccine should be approved. For example, the **FDA's Vaccines and Related Biological Products Advisory Committee (VRBPAC)** provides expert guidance on vaccine approval.

- **Risk-Benefit Analysis**: One of the primary responsibilities of regulatory authorities is to weigh the benefits of the vaccine (such as disease prevention) against any potential risks (such as side effects or adverse reactions). This analysis is crucial in determining whether the vaccine should be authorized for emergency use or full approval.

3. Emergency Use Authorization (EUA)

In cases where a vaccine is urgently needed, such as during an outbreak or a public health emergency, regulatory agencies can issue an **Emergency Use Authorization (EUA)**. An EUA allows a vaccine to be used before it has completed all the typical stages of clinical trials or when data is limited, but it still appears to offer substantial benefits in preventing the disease.

- **FDA and EUA**: In the United States, the FDA can grant an EUA for vaccines during emergencies like the COVID-19 pandemic. The vaccine must show that it meets certain criteria, such as demonstrating efficacy in preventing disease and a favorable safety profile in early-stage trials.

- **Global Response**: Other regulatory agencies, such as the EMA and WHO, can also grant similar emergency approvals for vaccines that meet the necessary criteria during public health emergencies.

4. Post-Market Surveillance: Ongoing Safety Monitoring

Even after a vaccine is approved and distributed, regulatory agencies continue to monitor its safety and effectiveness in the real world through post-market surveillance systems. These systems are designed to detect any adverse events or rare side effects that may not have been apparent during clinical trials.

- **Vaccine Adverse Event Reporting Systems (VAERS)**: In the United States, VAERS is a national system where healthcare providers, vaccine manufacturers, and the public can report adverse events following vaccination. The FDA and the CDC use VAERS data to monitor the safety of vaccines and investigate potential concerns.

- **Vaccine Safety Datalink (VSD)**: The CDC and the FDA collaborate on the VSD project, which uses data from large healthcare organizations to track and analyze the safety of vaccines in the population. This helps identify any potential long-term or rare side effects.

- **Global Monitoring**: Internationally, the WHO and other health agencies maintain global vaccine safety surveillance systems to track vaccine safety in various populations. The WHO's **Global Individual Case Safety Reports (ICSR)** provide data on adverse events reported globally.

5. Risk Communication and Transparency

Regulatory bodies must communicate clearly and transparently with the public about the benefits and risks of vaccines. This is essential in building trust in vaccination programs and ensuring that people are informed when making decisions about vaccination.

- **Public Health Guidance**: Health authorities issue guidance on vaccine safety and effectiveness based on the most current data. This may include updates on vaccine recommendations, addressing any new safety concerns, or providing guidance on the use of vaccines in specific populations.

- **Clear Labeling**: Regulatory agencies require vaccine manufacturers to provide clear and concise labeling, which includes information about the vaccine's ingredients, usage instructions, and potential side effects. This helps healthcare providers and patients make informed decisions.

- **Public Education Campaigns**: Health authorities often engage in public education campaigns to provide accurate information about vaccines and combat misinformation. This includes addressing common misconceptions, explaining the benefits of vaccination, and encouraging people to get vaccinated.

6. The Role of Regulatory Authorities in Global Vaccine Access

Regulatory agencies play a key role in ensuring that vaccines are accessible worldwide, particularly in low- and middle-income countries where access to vaccines can be limited. International organizations like the **WHO** and **GAVI, the Vaccine Alliance**, work to increase vaccine availability and ensure that vaccines are both affordable and safe for global populations.

- **Vaccine Prequalification**: The WHO prequalifies vaccines to ensure that they meet global safety and quality standards. This process helps facilitate the procurement of vaccines for use in global immunization programs.

- **Partnerships for Access**: Regulatory authorities work with governments, international organizations, and vaccine manufacturers to facilitate the distribution of vaccines in underserved areas. This includes working to ensure that vaccines are produced at scale and can reach remote or economically disadvantaged populations.

Conclusion

Regulatory authorities are vital to ensuring that vaccines are safe, effective, and of high quality. From the initial stages of vaccine development to post-market surveillance, these agencies oversee every aspect of the vaccine approval process, working to protect public health and promote the safe use of vaccines. Their role in risk assessment, transparency, and global access is essential in maintaining public trust in vaccination programs and ensuring that vaccines continue to save lives worldwide.

How Vaccine Safety Is Monitored Post-Market

Once a vaccine has been approved and made available to the public, its safety continues to be closely monitored. Post-market safety monitoring is a crucial part of the vaccine lifecycle, ensuring that any potential risks or side effects that were not apparent during clinical trials are detected early and addressed swiftly. This ongoing surveillance is necessary to maintain public trust in vaccination programs and to ensure that the benefits of vaccines continue to outweigh any potential risks.

1. Post-Market Surveillance Systems

Post-market surveillance involves the collection and analysis of data on the safety and effectiveness of vaccines once they are in widespread use. Several systems and programs are designed to detect and monitor adverse events (side effects) associated with vaccines.

- **Vaccine Adverse Event Reporting System (VAERS)**: In the United States, VAERS is a vital tool for monitoring vaccine safety. It is a national system run by the **Centers for Disease Control and Prevention (CDC)** and the **U.S. Food and Drug Administration (FDA)**. Healthcare providers, vaccine manufacturers, and the general public can report any adverse events (such as side effects or unexpected reactions) following vaccination. Although VAERS collects all reports, it does not confirm causality, but it is used to identify potential safety concerns that require further investigation.

- **Vaccine Safety Datalink (VSD)**: The CDC and FDA collaborate on the **Vaccine Safety Datalink**, a project that links data from large healthcare organizations, such as hospitals and insurance companies. The VSD tracks vaccine safety by monitoring health outcomes in populations that receive vaccines. This allows researchers to conduct in-depth studies to identify any rare or long-term adverse effects that might not have been seen in clinical trials.

- **Global Vaccine Safety Surveillance**: On a global scale, the **World Health Organization (WHO)** and national health authorities work together to monitor vaccine safety. The **Global Individual**

Case Safety Reports (ICSR) system enables countries to report adverse events to the WHO. This provides a comprehensive view of vaccine safety data across different regions and demographics, helping to identify any global concerns.

2. Types of Adverse Events Monitored

Post-market monitoring systems track a wide range of adverse events, including:

- **Common Side Effects**: These are expected and usually mild reactions to vaccines, such as soreness at the injection site, fever, or fatigue. These side effects are generally short-lived and are part of the body's natural immune response to the vaccine.

- **Serious Adverse Events (SAEs)**: Serious adverse events are rare but can include severe allergic reactions (anaphylaxis), seizures, or long-term health problems. Regulatory bodies investigate these events thoroughly to assess whether they were caused by the vaccine or are coincidental occurrences unrelated to the vaccination.

- **Uncommon or Rare Reactions**: Some side effects, though rare, may only be detected once the vaccine is administered to large populations. These include serious conditions like myocarditis (inflammation of the heart) or blood clotting disorders, which may be identified through post-market surveillance programs.

3. Signal Detection and Analysis

When adverse events are reported, regulatory authorities conduct thorough investigations to assess whether a potential safety issue exists. This process is known as **signal detection**, which involves identifying patterns in the data that suggest a possible link between the vaccine and a specific health problem.

- **Data Mining**: Health agencies use advanced statistical techniques to search for patterns in the data that may indicate a higher incidence of certain adverse events following vaccination. If a pattern is detected, further studies may be initiated to determine if there is a causal relationship.

- **Causality Assessment**: Not all adverse events reported to post-market surveillance systems are necessarily caused by the vaccine. To assess causality, health authorities analyze factors like the timing of the adverse event, the person's medical history, and the likelihood that the vaccine caused the reaction. This helps differentiate between events that are coincidental and those that may have been caused by the vaccine.

4. Ongoing Safety Monitoring and Communication

As part of post-market safety monitoring, regulatory agencies not only track adverse events but also provide continuous updates to the public and healthcare providers.

- **Safety Reviews and Updates**: Health authorities regularly review new safety data and update vaccine guidelines accordingly. For example, the CDC and FDA may issue new recommendations or safety alerts if new information emerges about the risks or benefits of a vaccine. These updates help ensure that healthcare providers and the public have the latest information on vaccine safety.

- **Risk Communication**: Effective communication is key in managing public perception of vaccine safety. Regulatory bodies work to provide clear and transparent information about the safety of vaccines, especially in response to any emerging concerns. This includes issuing public statements, conducting media outreach, and publishing safety reports that explain the risks and benefits of vaccines.

- **Vaccine Labeling and Warnings**: As part of the post-market process, vaccine manufacturers are required to update vaccine labeling and packaging with new safety information as it becomes available. This can include warnings about potential side effects or contraindications for specific groups, such as pregnant women or individuals with certain health conditions.

5. Long-Term Studies and Real-World Effectiveness

In addition to monitoring safety, post-market surveillance also includes ongoing studies to assess the **real-world effectiveness** of vaccines. These studies evaluate how well vaccines perform in the general population, including any variations in effectiveness across different groups (e.g., age, gender, or health conditions).

- **Real-World Data**: After vaccines are approved, real-world data provides important insights into their effectiveness in preventing disease under natural conditions. This includes monitoring how well a vaccine prevents infections, hospitalizations, and deaths in the broader population.

- **Post-Licensure Effectiveness Studies**: Health authorities may commission additional studies to track the effectiveness of vaccines over time, including any changes in the protection a vaccine provides against emerging variants or strains of a virus.

6. International Collaboration on Vaccine Safety

Vaccine safety is a global concern, and countries work together through international organizations like the **World Health Organization (WHO)** to ensure vaccines are safe and effective worldwide.

- **Global Surveillance Systems**: The WHO operates global surveillance systems to monitor vaccine safety and share information across countries. By pooling data from multiple countries, the WHO can identify safety signals and coordinate responses to potential concerns.

- **Vaccine Safety Initiatives**: The WHO's **Global Vaccine Safety Initiative** aims to strengthen national surveillance systems, improve the quality of safety data, and promote timely responses to adverse events. The initiative also works to improve public confidence in vaccines by providing evidence-based information on vaccine safety.

7. The Importance of Post-Market Surveillance in Building Trust

Post-market surveillance is a crucial part of maintaining the public's trust in vaccination programs. By continuously monitoring the safety of vaccines and transparently communicating findings, health authorities can address concerns and ensure that the benefits of vaccines continue to outweigh any potential risks. In addition, swift identification and response to safety issues are essential for protecting individuals and ensuring that vaccines remain a vital tool in preventing infectious diseases worldwide.

Conclusion

Post-market surveillance of vaccines is an ongoing, dynamic process that ensures vaccines remain safe and effective after they are approved for public use. Through robust reporting systems, real-time monitoring, and global collaboration, regulatory bodies can identify and address potential safety issues, provide updated information to healthcare providers and the public, and maintain confidence in the vaccination process. This vigilant approach helps ensure that vaccines continue to serve as one of the most powerful tools in safeguarding global health.

Chapter 3: The Vaccine Safety Debate

Vaccines have been pivotal in preventing infectious diseases and protecting public health. However, despite the overwhelming evidence of their safety and effectiveness, there are still several concerns that are frequently raised by individuals questioning vaccine safety. In this section, we will address some of the most common concerns, offering a detailed explanation based on scientific evidence to clarify the facts.

1. Vaccines and Autism: Dispelling the Myth

One of the most persistent and widely circulated concerns regarding vaccines is the belief that they cause autism. This misconception can be traced back to a 1998 study by British doctor Andrew Wakefield, which suggested a link between the MMR (measles, mumps, rubella) vaccine and autism. However, this study was thoroughly discredited, and Wakefield was later found guilty of scientific misconduct and had his medical license revoked. Numerous large-scale studies have since been conducted, all of which have found no connection between vaccines and autism.

- **The Evidence**: Studies involving large populations, such as one conducted in Denmark that included over 650,000 children, found no increased risk of autism in children who received the MMR vaccine. Similarly, the CDC and the World Health Organization (WHO) have consistently affirmed that vaccines, including the MMR vaccine, are not linked to autism.

- **Why This Concern Persists**: The enduring belief in the vaccine-autism link is largely due to misinformation and fear, as well as the emotional impact of autism diagnoses. However, research has repeatedly demonstrated that vaccines are not the cause, and the incidence of autism has increased regardless of vaccine coverage rates.

2. Vaccine Ingredients: Are They Safe?

Another common concern revolves around the ingredients used in vaccines. Some individuals worry about substances such as thimerosal, aluminum, formaldehyde, and other components found in vaccines, fearing that these could be harmful to health.

- **Thimerosal**: Thimerosal is a mercury-based preservative that was used in some vaccines. However, it has been removed from most childhood vaccines in the U.S. as a precautionary measure, even though scientific studies have shown that the levels of thimerosal used were too low to pose any risk. The only vaccines that still contain thimerosal in trace amounts are some flu vaccines, and there is no credible evidence linking thimerosal to harm.

- **Aluminum**: Aluminum is used in some vaccines as an adjuvant, which helps enhance the immune response. While high levels of aluminum can be toxic, the amount used in vaccines is far below harmful levels. The human body naturally processes small amounts of aluminum, and the levels in vaccines are considered safe by health authorities, including the CDC and WHO.

- **Formaldehyde**: Formaldehyde is used in vaccines to inactivate viruses or bacteria. It is found in very small quantities, much lower than what is typically present in the human body. The body uses formaldehyde as part of normal metabolic processes, and the levels used in vaccines are far below any toxic threshold.

- **Other Vaccine Ingredients**: The other ingredients used in vaccines, such as stabilizers and preservatives, are thoroughly tested for safety. Vaccines undergo rigorous safety assessments to ensure that their ingredients do not pose any harm to individuals receiving them.

3. Vaccine Overload: Is Too Many Vaccines Too Much for Children?

Some parents worry that receiving multiple vaccines in a short time could overwhelm their child's immune system. This concern is often referred to as "vaccine overload" or "immune system overload."

- **The Immune System's Capacity**: In reality, the immune system is capable of handling a far greater number of antigens (the parts of a virus or bacteria that trigger an immune response) than vaccines introduce. For example, a child's immune system encounters thousands of antigens every day from bacteria and viruses in their environment. Vaccines introduce only a tiny fraction of this total antigen load, and the immune system can effectively respond to all of them.

- **Vaccination Schedules**: Vaccination schedules are carefully designed to provide immunity against potentially deadly diseases at the appropriate times. The U.S. Centers for Disease Control and Prevention (CDC) and the American Academy of Pediatrics (AAP) recommend vaccines based on when they are most effective and when a child's immune system is ready to handle them. Spacing out vaccines or delaying them can leave children vulnerable to preventable diseases.

- **No Evidence of Harm**: There is no evidence to support the idea that receiving multiple vaccines at once harms the immune system or causes long-term health issues. On the contrary, by following the recommended vaccination schedule, children are protected from serious diseases as early as possible, offering the best chance for optimal health.

4. Vaccine Side Effects: Are They Dangerous?

Like any medical intervention, vaccines can cause side effects, but the vast majority are mild and temporary. These include reactions such as soreness at the injection site, low-grade fever, or fatigue. More severe side effects are extremely rare, and the benefits of vaccination far outweigh the risks of these minor reactions.

- **Common Side Effects**: The most common side effects of vaccines are mild and transient. These can include redness or swelling at the injection site, fever, and fatigue. These side effects typically resolve within a few days and are usually a sign that the immune system is responding to the vaccine.

- **Serious Side Effects**: Serious adverse reactions, such as severe allergic reactions (anaphylaxis), are rare, occurring in about 1 in a million doses for most vaccines. Health professionals are trained to recognize and manage any severe allergic reactions immediately, and vaccination clinics are equipped to handle emergencies.

- **Monitoring Vaccine Safety**: Vaccine safety is closely monitored through systems like VAERS (Vaccine Adverse Event Reporting System) in the U.S., which tracks any adverse events following vaccination. If any potential safety concerns arise, health authorities investigate to determine whether the vaccine caused the issue and take appropriate action if necessary.

5. The Role of Vaccines in Preventing Disease

One of the most compelling arguments in favor of vaccines is their effectiveness in preventing serious diseases. Vaccines have played a crucial role in eradicating smallpox and drastically reducing the prevalence of diseases like polio, measles, and diphtheria.

- **Herd Immunity**: Vaccines not only protect individuals who receive them but also help protect communities as a whole. When enough people are vaccinated against a contagious disease, it becomes harder for the disease to spread, offering protection to those who cannot be vaccinated, such as individuals with weakened immune systems or allergies to vaccine components.

- **The Impact of Vaccine Hesitancy**: Vaccine hesitancy, or the refusal to vaccinate, has contributed to outbreaks of preventable diseases. For example, the U.S. has seen a resurgence of measles, a disease that was nearly eradicated, due to declining vaccination rates. The World Health Organization (WHO) has identified vaccine hesitancy as one of the top 10 threats to global health, emphasizing the importance of continued vaccination efforts.

6. Vaccines and the Immune System: Will They Weaken It?

Another common concern is that vaccines might weaken the immune system, making individuals more susceptible to infections in the future. This is a misconception.

- **Strengthening, Not Weakening, Immunity**: Vaccines work by stimulating the immune system to produce a response against a specific pathogen, allowing the body to recognize and fight the pathogen if it encounters it in the future. Rather than weakening the immune system, vaccines help to "train" the immune system, making it more effective at recognizing and combating real infections.

- **Natural Immunity vs. Vaccine-Induced Immunity**: Some individuals believe that natural immunity, acquired by getting the disease, is superior to vaccine-induced immunity. However, natural infections can come with serious risks and complications, such as hospitalization or long-term health effects. Vaccination provides a safe and controlled way to develop immunity without the risks associated with contracting the disease itself.

Conclusion

While concerns about vaccine safety are common, the evidence supporting the safety and effectiveness of vaccines is overwhelming. Vaccines save lives, prevent disease, and protect the most vulnerable members of society. It is essential to address misconceptions, provide accurate information, and continue to promote trust in vaccines to ensure that everyone can benefit from their protective power. The scientific community, public health experts, and global health organizations are committed to maintaining the safety of vaccines, ensuring that their benefits continue to outweigh any potential risks.

Vaccine Adverse Events: How Real Are the Risks?

accine adverse events (AEs) are an important aspect of public health discussions, as they pertain to any side effects or reactions that occur following vaccination. It's crucial to understand the nature, frequency, and severity of these events to assess the real risks associated with vaccines. This section will delve into the science behind vaccine-related adverse events, their actual risks, and how they are monitored and managed.

1. Understanding Vaccine Adverse Events

A vaccine adverse event refers to any unintended or undesirable health effect that occurs after receiving a vaccine. These events can range from mild, short-term side effects to rare, serious reactions. It's important to differentiate between reactions that are directly caused by the vaccine and those that may happen coincidentally after vaccination.

- **Types of Adverse Events**: Adverse events are classified into two categories:

  - **Local Reactions**: These occur at the site of the injection, such as redness, swelling, or pain. These reactions are typically mild and resolve within a few days.

  - **Systemic Reactions**: These affect the body more broadly and can include fever, fatigue, headache, and muscle aches. These side effects are often short-lived and a sign that the body is building immunity.

- **Serious Adverse Events**: In rare cases, individuals may experience more severe reactions, such as anaphylaxis (a severe allergic reaction) or Guillain-Barré syndrome (a rare neurological condition). However, these serious events are exceedingly rare and are typically well-managed by healthcare providers.

2. Frequency of Vaccine Adverse Events

The vast majority of people who receive vaccines do not experience any adverse events, and for those who do, the reactions are usually mild and temporary. According to data from various public health organizations, the incidence of serious vaccine-related adverse events is extremely low.

- **Mild Adverse Events**: These are very common and can include swelling or tenderness at the injection site, low-grade fever, or temporary tiredness. Such reactions usually resolve within a day or two and are considered a normal part of the body's immune response.

- **Serious Adverse Events**: Serious adverse events, such as anaphylaxis or long-term disabilities, are rare. For example, the rate of anaphylaxis from vaccines is about 1 in a million doses for most vaccines, according to the U.S. Centers for Disease Control and Prevention (CDC). In the case of the MMR vaccine, studies have shown no significant increased risk of Guillain-Barré syndrome.

3. Risk vs. Benefit: Evaluating Vaccine Safety

While no medical intervention is entirely without risk, vaccines are thoroughly tested for safety before being approved for public use. The risks associated with vaccines are small in comparison to the benefits they provide in preventing serious diseases, hospitalizations, and deaths.

- **Vaccine Safety Monitoring**: Vaccine safety is rigorously monitored through various systems such as the Vaccine Adverse Event Reporting System (VAERS) in the U.S. This system allows healthcare providers and the public to report any adverse events following vaccination. The data collected from VAERS is used to detect potential safety signals, investigate the cause of these events, and determine whether further action is needed, such as revising vaccine recommendations or improving vaccine formulations.

- **The Benefit of Immunization**: Vaccines prevent the spread of contagious and sometimes deadly diseases. Diseases like polio, measles, and diphtheria, which once caused widespread illness and death, have been dramatically reduced due to global vaccination efforts. The benefits of immunization—such as herd immunity, protection for vulnerable populations, and the eradication of diseases—far outweigh the rare risks of adverse events.

- **Public Health Impact**: The benefits of vaccines extend beyond the individual, contributing to public health by reducing disease transmission and providing indirect protection to those who cannot receive vaccines, such as infants too young for certain immunizations or individuals with compromised immune systems.

4. Investigating and Responding to Serious Adverse Events

When serious adverse events occur, they are thoroughly investigated by health authorities. These investigations involve determining whether the vaccine caused the event or whether it was coincidental. In many cases, a causal relationship is not found, and the adverse event is determined to be unrelated to the vaccine. However, when a potential link is discovered, health agencies can take appropriate actions to mitigate future risks, such as modifying vaccine guidelines or recommending additional precautions.

- **Anaphylaxis**: This severe allergic reaction is one of the most frequently discussed serious adverse events associated with vaccines. However, anaphylaxis is extremely rare, and healthcare providers are trained to manage it immediately if it occurs. People who have a history of severe allergic reactions to any vaccine ingredient are typically advised not to receive that vaccine.

- **The Role of Monitoring**: After vaccines are approved for use, they continue to be monitored in the real world. This post-marketing surveillance is essential to ensure that any rare adverse events that might not have been detected during clinical trials are identified and addressed. If a rare adverse event is detected, steps are taken to protect public health, such as revising vaccine recommendations or issuing public health alerts.

5. How Health Authorities Manage Vaccine Safety

Health authorities, including the CDC, the World Health Organization (WHO), and the U.S. Food and Drug Administration (FDA), play critical roles in ensuring that vaccines remain safe after they are approved for use. They utilize a combination of pre-approval clinical trials, real-world surveillance, and post-market monitoring to assess the ongoing safety of vaccines.

- **Clinical Trials**: Before a vaccine is licensed, it undergoes extensive testing in clinical trials, which are designed to identify any potential risks. These trials are conducted in multiple phases, with each phase designed to gather information about the vaccine's safety, effectiveness, and potential side effects.

- **Post-Marketing Surveillance**: Once a vaccine is authorized for use, surveillance systems like VAERS and the Vaccine Safety Datalink (VSD) continue to monitor for any adverse events that may occur in the general population. If any safety concerns arise, health authorities investigate these incidents and take appropriate action to ensure that the benefits of vaccination continue to outweigh any risks.

- **Global Vaccine Safety**: The WHO, in addition to overseeing vaccine safety in individual countries, also works to ensure that vaccines meet international safety standards. This includes coordinating global vaccination efforts and responding to any emerging vaccine safety concerns.

6. Addressing Public Concerns: Education and Transparency

Public trust in vaccines is essential for maintaining high vaccination rates and protecting population health. To build and maintain this trust, it is crucial that health authorities, healthcare providers, and scientists remain transparent about vaccine safety, provide accurate information, and address concerns directly.

- **Clear Communication**: Addressing the risks of vaccines with clear, transparent information helps demystify potential adverse events. By providing factual, evidence-based information, health authorities can reassure the public about the rarity of serious adverse events and the overwhelming benefits of vaccination.

- **Ongoing Research**: Research into vaccine safety is ongoing, with new studies being conducted regularly to ensure that vaccines remain safe as they are used by millions of people worldwide. Scientific advances continue to improve vaccine formulations and delivery methods, further reducing the risk of adverse events.

Conclusion: The Real Risks of Vaccines

While vaccine adverse events can occur, the risks are minimal compared to the significant benefits that vaccines offer. The overwhelming majority of people who receive vaccines experience no serious side effects, and any adverse events that do occur are generally mild and short-lived. Serious adverse events, such as anaphylaxis, are extremely rare and are closely monitored by healthcare professionals to ensure prompt and appropriate treatment.

Ultimately, vaccines have proven to be one of the most successful public health interventions in history, saving millions of lives and preventing countless cases of serious illness. By understanding the risks, monitoring safety, and continuing to communicate openly with the public, we can ensure that vaccines continue to play a central role in safeguarding global health.

The Role of the Vaccine Adverse Event Reporting System (VAERS)

The Vaccine Adverse Event Reporting System (VAERS) is a crucial tool in the ongoing process of monitoring vaccine safety. Managed by the U.S. Centers for Disease Control and Prevention (CDC) and the U.S. Food and Drug Administration (FDA), VAERS allows healthcare professionals, vaccine recipients, and caregivers to report any adverse events that occur after vaccination. This system plays a key role in detecting potential safety concerns and ensuring that vaccines remain safe and effective for the general population. Below, we explore the purpose, function, and impact of VAERS in more detail.

1. What is VAERS?

VAERS is a national system that collects and analyzes reports of adverse events (AEs) following vaccination. It serves as an early warning system to detect possible safety issues related to vaccines. The reports can be submitted by healthcare providers, vaccine recipients, and others who may notice a reaction after a person receives a vaccine.

- **Adverse Events**: These include any undesirable side effects, from mild reactions like sore arms or fever to more serious events like allergic reactions or neurological issues. The system also collects reports on events that may not be directly caused by the vaccine but happen after vaccination.

- **Voluntary Reporting**: While healthcare providers are encouraged to report AEs, the system also allows anyone (including patients and their families) to submit a report. This voluntary aspect ensures that all potential incidents are captured, even if the healthcare provider doesn't make the report themselves.

2. How Does VAERS Work?

VAERS works by collecting data on reported adverse events, regardless of whether or not the vaccine is definitively linked to the event. The system is intended to identify patterns or unusual occurrences that may warrant further investigation. Here's how the system functions:

- **Data Collection**: VAERS collects data on the type of vaccine administered, the adverse event that occurred, the timing of the reaction, the demographic information of the individual, and any other relevant details. This helps to create a comprehensive database of potential vaccine side effects.

- **Data Analysis**: The CDC and FDA analyze the data submitted to VAERS to identify trends and signals that may indicate a safety concern. For instance, if a large number of people report the same serious adverse event after receiving a specific vaccine, it could signal a potential problem that requires further research.

- **Signal Detection**: VAERS uses statistical methods to detect patterns that might indicate a potential link between a vaccine and an adverse event. If a particular vaccine is associated with an unexpected or unusually high rate of a specific adverse event, the system can trigger a more detailed investigation.

- **Follow-Up and Investigation**: When a signal is detected, VAERS data may prompt further investigation by health authorities. The CDC, FDA, and other organizations may conduct additional studies, look at clinical trial data, or perform risk-benefit analyses to better understand the situation. Based on these findings, vaccine recommendations may be adjusted if needed.

3. The Importance of VAERS in Vaccine Safety

VAERS plays an integral role in ensuring that vaccines are safe and effective. By acting as an early detection system for potential problems, VAERS helps public health authorities monitor and address vaccine safety in real-time. Here are the key ways that VAERS supports vaccine safety:

- **Early Detection of Rare Adverse Events**: Most adverse events associated with vaccines are mild and temporary, but some rare reactions may only become apparent once a vaccine is used widely across the population. VAERS provides a mechanism for identifying these rare events quickly.

- **Ongoing Safety Monitoring**: Even after a vaccine is licensed and widely used, VAERS continues to monitor for adverse events. This allows for long-term surveillance of the vaccine's safety profile. If any safety concerns arise after a vaccine is in use, VAERS provides the data needed to investigate and address those concerns promptly.

- **Transparency and Public Trust**: By allowing the public to report adverse events, VAERS helps to maintain transparency in the vaccination process. This openness ensures that individuals can trust the vaccine safety monitoring system and feel confident that their health concerns are being addressed.

4. Limitations of VAERS

While VAERS is an essential tool for vaccine safety surveillance, it does have some limitations:

- **Reporting Bias**: Since reporting to VAERS is voluntary, there may be biases in the data. Some adverse events may not be reported, and some reports may be exaggerated or unfounded. This can complicate the analysis and interpretation of the data.

- **Causality**: It's important to understand that VAERS reports do not prove causality. Just because an adverse event is reported after vaccination doesn't mean the vaccine caused the event. The system merely collects data and flags potential concerns, which must then be investigated through further research.

- **Incomplete Data**: In some cases, reports may lack detailed information, which can hinder thorough analysis. For instance, if there is insufficient data about the patient's medical history or the exact timing of the adverse event, it becomes difficult to draw definitive conclusions.

- **Focus on New Vaccines**: VAERS tends to focus more on new vaccines or vaccines with changing recommendations (such as during a public health emergency), which means some vaccines with longer histories may not receive the same level of attention unless an unusual trend is noticed.

5. VAERS vs. Other Vaccine Safety Monitoring Systems

VAERS is just one component of the broader vaccine safety monitoring system. There are other systems in place that complement VAERS, providing a more comprehensive safety evaluation:

- **Vaccine Safety Datalink (VSD)**: This system, managed by the CDC, uses data from several large healthcare organizations to monitor vaccine safety. Unlike VAERS, which relies on voluntary reporting, the VSD uses electronic health records to track vaccine side effects in real time. The VSD provides more detailed information and is used to conduct more in-depth studies.

- **Clinical Trials and Post-Licensure Studies**: Before a vaccine is approved for public use, it undergoes rigorous clinical trials to evaluate its safety. Post-licensure studies, such as cohort studies or randomized controlled trials, continue to monitor vaccines after approval to further assess long-term safety.

- **Global Vaccine Safety Monitoring**: The World Health Organization (WHO) and other international health bodies also monitor vaccine safety globally. These agencies rely on national health organizations and collaborate on global surveillance to ensure that vaccines are safe and effective worldwide.

6. Responding to Safety Signals and Addressing Public Concerns

When VAERS detects a potential safety issue, it triggers further investigation. Public health authorities take these signals seriously and investigate whether a particular vaccine is linked to the reported adverse event. If necessary, vaccine recommendations can be adjusted to protect public health.

- **Corrective Actions**: If an adverse event is deemed to be related to a vaccine, authorities may recommend specific actions such as revising dosing guidelines, changing the way the vaccine is administered, or even withdrawing the vaccine if the risks outweigh the benefits.

- **Educational Efforts**: Addressing concerns and providing clear, accurate information is essential for maintaining public trust in the vaccine safety monitoring process. Health authorities often work to educate the public on the findings from VAERS and other safety monitoring systems, explaining the risks and benefits of vaccines and offering reassurance.

Conclusion: The Vital Role of VAERS in Ensuring Vaccine Safety

The Vaccine Adverse Event Reporting System (VAERS) is an essential tool in the ongoing effort to monitor vaccine safety. By collecting and analyzing reports of adverse events, VAERS plays a critical role in identifying potential risks and ensuring that vaccines continue to provide benefits that outweigh the risks. While VAERS has some limitations, it remains a cornerstone of public health efforts to maintain vaccine safety, respond to concerns, and protect global health. Through systems like VAERS, the safety of vaccines is continuously scrutinized, allowing for quick responses to emerging safety signals and fostering greater public confidence in immunization programs.

Investigating Claims of Vaccine Injuries and the Role of Epidemiology

Investigating claims of vaccine injuries is a critical aspect of ensuring the safety and effectiveness of immunization programs. While vaccines are widely recognized for their role in preventing infectious diseases, occasional claims of adverse events following vaccination can raise concerns. Understanding how these claims are investigated and the role that epidemiology plays in this process is essential for clarifying the safety of vaccines and providing evidence-based answers to the public.

1. What Are Vaccine Injuries?

Vaccine injuries are adverse events that occur after vaccination and are sometimes claimed to be caused by the vaccine itself. These events can range from mild reactions like redness at the injection site, fever, or fatigue, to more severe conditions such as anaphylaxis, neurological disorders, or autoimmune reactions.

It is important to note that the vast majority of vaccine reactions are mild and temporary, and serious side effects are rare. However, the possibility of adverse events can lead to widespread debate and concerns, especially in cases where the cause of the injury is unclear.

2. Investigating Claims of Vaccine Injuries

When a claim of a vaccine injury is made, it is crucial to systematically investigate whether the vaccine actually caused the adverse event. This investigation typically involves several steps:

- **Initial Reporting**: The first step in the investigation process is the reporting of the adverse event, typically through systems like the Vaccine Adverse Event Reporting System (VAERS) or directly to healthcare providers. The individual reporting the event might be a healthcare professional, the person receiving the vaccine, or a caregiver.

- **Medical Review and Diagnosis**: Once a claim is reported, the next step involves medical professionals reviewing the individual's health history, the timing of the vaccination, and the nature of the adverse event. They assess whether the symptoms are consistent with known side effects of the vaccine, whether the event could be due to other underlying conditions, or if the timing of the event aligns with the expected response to vaccination.

- **Causality Assessment**: Determining whether a vaccine caused an injury is often complex. Many factors must be considered, including the individual's medical history, pre-existing conditions, other medications, and the timing of the event. A range of diagnostic tools, including lab tests, imaging, and patient history, may be used to rule out other potential causes.

3. The Role of Epidemiology in Investigating Vaccine Injuries

Epidemiology plays a crucial role in investigating and understanding claims of vaccine injuries. Epidemiologists use scientific methods to study patterns of disease, health events, and exposure to risk factors in populations. In the case of vaccine injuries, epidemiologists help determine whether there is an association between a vaccine and a particular adverse event, and if so, the strength and significance of that association.

- **Observational Studies**: Epidemiologists use observational studies, such as cohort studies and case-control studies, to assess whether people who receive a vaccine are more likely to experience certain adverse events compared to those who do not receive the vaccine. These studies look for patterns in large groups of people, often comparing vaccinated individuals with those who are unvaccinated or who received a different vaccine.

  - **Cohort Studies**: These studies follow two groups over time—those who receive the vaccine and those who do not—and monitor the occurrence of adverse events in both groups. This can help identify any increased risk of injury from vaccination.

- **Case-Control Studies**: In these studies, researchers compare individuals who experienced a specific adverse event (the "cases") with those who did not (the "controls") to see if vaccination or specific factors related to vaccination are more common in the injured group. This approach helps to identify potential links between vaccination and rare adverse events.

- **Data from Surveillance Systems**: Epidemiologists also rely on data from vaccine safety surveillance systems, such as VAERS, the Vaccine Safety Datalink (VSD), and the Clinical Immunization Safety Assessment (CISA) Network, to detect signals of possible adverse events. These systems collect large volumes of data on vaccine recipients, and epidemiologists analyze this data to identify trends, such as an unusually high incidence of a particular injury following a specific vaccine.

- **Risk-Benefit Analysis**: Epidemiologists play a key role in conducting risk-benefit analyses, which weigh the potential risks of a vaccine against its benefits. This analysis helps determine whether a vaccine's protective benefits outweigh any potential risks, particularly when it comes to rare adverse events. The results of these analyses are crucial for public health decision-making, as they guide recommendations for vaccine use.

4. Assessing Causality in Epidemiology

In epidemiology, determining causality—whether a vaccine directly causes a particular injury—requires rigorous evidence. Several criteria are used to assess causality in the context of vaccine injuries:

- **Temporality**: The timing of the adverse event is critical in determining causality. The event must occur within a reasonable time frame following vaccination. While some side effects are immediate, others may take weeks or months to manifest.

- **Consistency**: If similar adverse events are repeatedly observed in vaccinated individuals, it strengthens the case for causality. However, if an adverse event is rare and isolated, it may indicate that the cause is unrelated to the vaccine.

- **Biological Plausibility**: The biological mechanism behind a potential vaccine injury is an important consideration. Epidemiologists and immunologists work together to determine whether there is a plausible biological explanation for how a vaccine could cause the alleged injury. For example, some vaccines may trigger autoimmune reactions in predisposed individuals, but such cases are very rare.

- **Strength of the Association**: A strong association between vaccination and the injury is more likely to indicate a causal link. However, even a strong association may not be sufficient to prove causality, especially if other factors, such as genetics or pre-existing conditions, contribute to the event.

- **Specificity**: If the injury is specific to a particular vaccine or group of people, this may indicate a stronger causal link. However, vaccines are tested across diverse populations, and specific adverse events are often rare.

- **Reversibility**: If the adverse event resolves after discontinuation of vaccination or medical intervention, it can support a causal link between the vaccine and the injury. Conversely, if the injury persists despite treatment, it may suggest an alternative cause.

5. Addressing Public Concerns and Communication

When claims of vaccine injuries arise, it is essential for public health authorities to provide clear and transparent information. Epidemiological studies and evidence-based findings are crucial in addressing public concerns and promoting trust in the vaccine safety monitoring process. Here are some key strategies for effective communication:

- **Clear Communication of Findings**: Health authorities must communicate the results of epidemiological investigations in a clear and accessible manner. This includes sharing both the benefits and risks of vaccines in a way that the general public can understand. Transparency about the investigative process helps build trust in the safety of vaccines.

- **Public Education on Vaccine Safety**: Ongoing public education campaigns about vaccine safety and the risks of vaccine-preventable diseases can help to mitigate concerns about potential vaccine injuries. These campaigns can also help to clarify misconceptions about the risks and benefits of vaccines, reducing vaccine hesitancy.

- **Engagement with Affected Individuals**: When a vaccine injury is claimed, engaging with the affected individual and providing support is essential. Health professionals should ensure that individuals are properly diagnosed, receive appropriate medical care, and are given a fair hearing if they believe they have been harmed by a vaccine.

- **Post-Vaccination Support Systems**: Providing clear pathways for individuals to report adverse events and seek compensation, such as through the National Vaccine Injury Compensation Program (VICP), helps address concerns and ensures that those affected by potential vaccine injuries are supported.

6. Conclusion: The Importance of Rigorous Investigation and Epidemiology

Investigating claims of vaccine injuries is a complex and important process that requires careful attention to scientific evidence, patient history, and epidemiological data. Epidemiology plays a vital role in determining whether a vaccine is causally linked to an adverse event and in understanding the broader context of vaccine safety. By using a rigorous, evidence-based approach, we can better understand the risks and benefits of vaccination, address public concerns, and ensure that immunization programs continue to protect public health while minimizing harm.

Chapter 4: Myths and Misconceptions About Vaccines

Myth #1: Vaccines Cause Autism

One of the most persistent and harmful myths surrounding vaccines is the belief that they cause autism, particularly the claim that the MMR (measles, mumps, rubella) vaccine is linked to the development of autism spectrum disorder (ASD). This myth has had a significant impact on vaccine hesitancy, leading to increased fear among parents and communities about the safety of immunization.

The Origin of the Myth

The myth can be traced back to a 1998 study published by Andrew Wakefield, a British former doctor, in *The Lancet*, a prestigious medical journal. In this study, Wakefield claimed to have found a link between the MMR vaccine and autism in children. His study, which involved only 12 children, suggested that the vaccine caused gastrointestinal problems that, in turn, led to the development of autism.

However, the study was deeply flawed. Later investigations revealed serious ethical issues, such as undisclosed financial conflicts of interest and manipulation of data. The study was retracted in 2010, and Wakefield lost his medical license due to his fraudulent research practices. Despite this, the damage was done, and the myth that vaccines cause autism persisted.

The Reality: No Evidence of a Link

Since the publication and retraction of Wakefield's study, numerous large-scale, well-conducted studies have been carried out to investigate whether there is any association between vaccines and autism. The overwhelming consensus among scientists and health experts is that there is no link between vaccines, including the MMR vaccine, and autism.

- **Scientific Studies**: A landmark study published in 2019 in the *Annals of Internal Medicine* followed over 650,000 children and found no increased risk of autism in those who received the MMR vaccine compared to those who did not. This study is just one of many that have been conducted over the past two decades, all of which consistently show no connection between vaccines and autism.

- **Further Research**: Studies have examined various aspects of vaccine safety, including the timing of vaccine administration and the number of vaccines given to children. All have concluded that there is no evidence to support the idea that vaccines cause autism. For instance, a large study published in *JAMA* (Journal of the American Medical Association) in 2015 reviewed more than 95,000 children and found no increased risk of autism with the MMR vaccine.

Why the Myth Endures

Despite the wealth of scientific evidence disproving the link between vaccines and autism, the myth continues to spread. Several factors contribute to this:

- **Confirmation Bias**: People who believe in the vaccine-autism link may be more likely to seek out information that supports their beliefs, even if that information is inaccurate or misleading.

- **Influence of Anti-Vaccine Groups**: Anti-vaccine groups have played a significant role in perpetuating the myth by spreading misinformation online and in social media. These groups often use emotional appeals and anecdotes to fuel fears, rather than relying on scientific evidence.

- **The Appeal of Causality**: Autism diagnoses have increased in recent decades, and some parents may be searching for a cause or explanation. The timing of the MMR vaccine, which is given around the same time that children are often diagnosed with autism, has led to a false assumption that the two are connected.

The Importance of Vaccination

Vaccines, including the MMR vaccine, have been shown to be safe, effective, and essential in preventing serious diseases. Measles, mumps, and rubella are all highly contagious diseases that can cause severe complications, including pneumonia, encephalitis (brain inflammation), hearing loss, and even death. The MMR vaccine provides critical protection against these diseases, and the risks of not vaccinating far outweigh the unfounded fears about autism.

- **Herd Immunity**: Vaccination not only protects the individual but also helps protect vulnerable populations who cannot be vaccinated, such as infants, pregnant women, and those with weakened immune systems. When a large percentage of the population is vaccinated, it creates herd immunity, preventing outbreaks and ensuring that diseases remain under control.

Conclusion

The myth that vaccines cause autism has been thoroughly debunked by science. No credible research supports this claim, and the overwhelming evidence indicates that vaccines are safe and essential in preventing infectious diseases. It is crucial for individuals, especially parents, to seek information from reputable sources, such as public health organizations and scientific studies, rather than relying on misinformation from anti-vaccine advocates. By debunking this myth and others, we can ensure that vaccines continue to be a vital tool in protecting public health and preventing the spread of harmful diseases.

Myth #2: Vaccines Overwhelm the Immune System

Another common misconception about vaccines is that they "overwhelm" the immune system, especially in infants and young children, who receive multiple vaccines as part of their routine immunization schedule. Many people fear that the body cannot handle the number of antigens present in vaccines and that this may lead to immune system dysfunction or harm. However, this myth is based on a misunderstanding of how the immune system works and how vaccines function.

The Origin of the Myth

This myth likely arose from concerns about the number of vaccines given to children, particularly the increasing number of vaccines added to the childhood immunization schedule in recent decades. As new vaccines were developed and recommended for various diseases, some individuals expressed concern that the sheer number of vaccinations would be too much for a child's developing immune system to manage.

The Reality: The Immune System Can Handle Far More Than Vaccines Expose It To

In reality, the immune system is incredibly sophisticated and capable of handling far more challenges than vaccines present. Here's why the myth that vaccines overwhelm the immune system is not true:

- **Immune System Capacity**: The human immune system is constantly exposed to a vast array of pathogens, from bacteria to viruses, every day. In fact, it can handle and respond to millions of different pathogens. When you encounter germs in the environment (like when you touch surfaces or breathe in air), your immune system is already in action, defending your body from infection.

Vaccines are a tiny fraction of what the immune system deals with on a daily basis. The number of antigens in all the vaccines a child receives in their first few years of life is a small fraction of the number their immune system is exposed to in their everyday environment.

- **Antigens in Vaccines**: An antigen is any substance that triggers an immune response, and vaccines contain only a small part of a virus or bacterium, such as a protein or inactivated version of the pathogen. The idea that vaccines contain a large number of antigens and therefore burden the immune system is misleading. For example, while children may receive several vaccines at once, the total number of antigens in all those vaccines is far fewer than the number of antigens their body is exposed to through common viruses, bacteria, and even harmless substances like pollen.

- **Safe and Effective Schedules**: The recommended vaccination schedule has been designed carefully by public health experts, including the Centers for Disease Control and Prevention (CDC) and the World Health Organization (WHO), to ensure that vaccines are given at the most appropriate times in a child's development. These schedules allow the immune system to respond to vaccines without overloading it. The schedule is based on years of research and testing and ensures that the immune system is not overwhelmed while providing the best protection possible against potentially dangerous diseases.

- **A Drop in Disease Incidence**: Thanks to vaccines, we have seen dramatic reductions in the incidence of many diseases that were once common and deadly, such as measles, polio, and whooping cough. The vaccines that protect against these diseases have undergone rigorous testing and are proven to be both safe and effective. In fact, the routine use of vaccines has saved millions of lives globally by preventing outbreaks of diseases that can cause severe complications or death.

How Vaccines Stimulate the Immune System

When a vaccine is administered, it presents a harmless piece or version of the pathogen (often a protein or inactivated virus) to the immune system. This allows the body to mount a response, which includes the production of antibodies that are specifically tailored to recognize and fight that pathogen if encountered again in the future. This process is both highly efficient and controlled by the immune system's sophisticated mechanisms, and it does not "overwhelm" the immune system in any way.

- **Memory Cells**: After vaccination, the immune system "remembers" how to fight the disease if exposed to it in the future. This immune memory is one of the key benefits of vaccination. It means that the body can recognize and fight the pathogen more quickly and effectively if it encounters it again.

- **Simultaneous Vaccination**: It's important to note that children are often given multiple vaccines during a single visit to the doctor. This might include vaccines for diseases such as polio, diphtheria, tetanus, pertussis, and others. This is not an issue for the immune system because the body has the ability to manage multiple immune responses at once. The immune system can handle a variety of pathogens and vaccines simultaneously without difficulty.

The Myth in Perspective: How Many Antigens Can the Immune System Handle?

One of the common concerns about vaccines is the idea that the number of antigens in the full set of childhood vaccinations might be too much for the immune system. The reality is that even if a child received all the recommended vaccines at once, their immune system would still have the capacity to handle many more antigens than those found in the vaccines.

- **The Immunological Load**: In total, the childhood vaccination schedule exposes a child to only about 150-200 antigens (depending on the number of vaccines given). By comparison, just one common cold virus contains 10,000 to 100,000 different antigens. So, the immune system is routinely challenged with much larger numbers of antigens from everyday exposure to bacteria and viruses in the environment.

- **The Safety of Multiple Vaccines**: Studies have shown that receiving multiple vaccines in a single visit is safe and does not overwhelm the immune system. In fact, research comparing children who receive vaccines on the recommended schedule versus those who are delayed or skip vaccines has shown no difference in immune system function, confirming that the recommended schedule is both safe and optimal for protection.

The Role of Vaccination in Public Health

Vaccines not only protect individuals but also protect the broader community by reducing the spread of infectious diseases. This is particularly important for vulnerable populations, such as newborns, the elderly, and individuals with weakened immune systems, who may not be able to receive certain vaccines themselves. Vaccines ensure that diseases remain under control, preventing outbreaks and saving lives.

Conclusion

The myth that vaccines overwhelm the immune system is not supported by science. Vaccines are a safe and effective way to protect individuals and communities from dangerous diseases, and the immune system is more than capable of handling the number of antigens found in the recommended vaccination schedule. Understanding the true capacity of the immune system and the science behind vaccines is essential in dispelling this myth and ensuring that everyone can make informed decisions about vaccination.

Myth #3: Natural Immunity Is Better Than Vaccine-Induced Immunity

One of the most common myths in the vaccine debate is the belief that natural immunity — immunity gained through recovering from an infection — is superior to immunity provided by vaccines. While it's true that natural immunity can provide protection after an infection, this myth fails to consider several important factors, including the risks associated with getting sick, the consistency and reliability of vaccine-induced immunity, and the broader public health benefits of vaccination.

The Origin of the Myth

The myth that natural immunity is better than vaccine-induced immunity likely stems from the historical reliance on natural infection for immune protection. Before vaccines were developed, people had no choice but to rely on natural infection to build immunity against many diseases. This led to the belief that immunity gained through a natural infection was somehow more "authentic" or stronger.

However, with the advancement of vaccine science, this myth has been debunked, and it is now well understood that vaccines provide a safe and reliable way to achieve immunity without exposing individuals to the harmful effects of illness.

Why Natural Immunity Isn't Always Better

1. **Risk of Severe Illness:**

    o   Natural infection often leads to illness, and in many cases, it can result in severe complications, hospitalization, or even death. For example, diseases like measles, chickenpox, and whooping cough can be life-threatening, especially for young children, the elderly, and those with weakened immune systems. Natural infection may provide immunity, but it comes with significant health risks, including long-term complications such as brain damage, lung damage, or infertility.

    o   In contrast, vaccines allow people to gain immunity without having to experience the full-blown disease. Vaccines stimulate the immune system in a controlled and safe manner, avoiding the dangers of the disease itself.

2. **Variability of Natural Immunity:**

    o   Natural immunity can vary greatly from person to person. Some individuals may develop robust immunity after recovering from an infection, while others may have weaker immune responses. This variability can leave certain individuals at risk for reinfection.

    o   In contrast, vaccines are designed to produce a consistent and controlled immune response in the vast majority of recipients, making them a more reliable way to prevent infection.

3. **Duration of Immunity**:

   - Immunity gained through natural infection does not always last as long as immunity provided by vaccines. For some diseases, the immune protection from a natural infection can wane over time, leaving individuals susceptible to reinfection years later. For example, natural immunity to diseases like pertussis (whooping cough) or influenza may diminish over time, while vaccine-induced immunity may be boosted with additional doses, ensuring longer-lasting protection.

   - Many vaccines, such as those for measles or diphtheria, provide long-lasting immunity with very few booster shots, allowing individuals to maintain immunity without the need to experience the disease again.

4. **Herd Immunity and Community Protection**:

   - Vaccination is not just about protecting the individual; it's also about protecting the community. When enough people are vaccinated, it creates herd immunity, which helps protect those who cannot receive vaccines due to medical reasons (such as allergies or weakened immune systems) or those who are too young to be vaccinated.

- o Natural infection does not contribute to herd immunity in the same way. In fact, allowing large numbers of people to become infected can actually spread disease and endanger vulnerable populations. Vaccination, on the other hand, contributes to community-wide immunity by preventing the spread of infection.

5. **The Power of Vaccines in Preventing Outbreaks**:

- o The success of vaccines in preventing widespread outbreaks of diseases like smallpox, polio, and more recently, COVID-19, demonstrates the power of vaccine-induced immunity. Diseases that were once widespread and deadly are now rare or eradicated because vaccines have provided a safe, reliable, and scalable way to protect populations.

- o Natural immunity alone cannot achieve the same effect on a population-wide level. The goal of vaccination is to prevent outbreaks and ensure that the entire population is protected, reducing the spread of infectious diseases.

Comparing Natural Immunity and Vaccine-Induced Immunity

- **Strength of Immunity**: While natural infection often produces a strong immune response, vaccines are designed to simulate the same response without causing illness. For many diseases, vaccine-induced immunity is just as effective, if not more effective, than natural immunity. For instance, the immunity gained from the measles vaccine is both strong and long-lasting, similar to immunity gained from a natural infection, but without the risk of complications from the disease itself.

- **Speed of Immunity**: With vaccines, immunity is achieved much more quickly and safely than through natural infection. For example, the COVID-19 vaccines provide protection against the virus within a matter of weeks, while natural immunity can take longer to develop and comes with a higher risk of illness during the process.

- **Boosters and Updates**: Vaccines can be updated and refined over time to provide better protection against evolving strains of a virus. For example, the flu vaccine is updated annually to account for changes in circulating flu strains, while natural immunity may not offer the same level of protection against new variants of a disease.

The Role of Vaccines in Public Health

Vaccination programs have been pivotal in reducing the burden of infectious diseases globally. Thanks to vaccines, many diseases that once caused widespread illness and death, such as polio, smallpox, and rubella, have been significantly reduced or eradicated. In many cases, vaccines offer a safer and more reliable way to protect individuals and the public from these diseases than natural immunity ever could.

Conclusion

The myth that natural immunity is always better than vaccine-induced immunity overlooks the risks associated with natural infection, the variability of immune responses, and the broader public health benefits of vaccination. While natural immunity may provide protection, vaccines offer a safer, more controlled, and reliable means of achieving immunity without the dangers of disease. Vaccination not only protects individuals but also contributes to community-wide immunity, ensuring that vulnerable populations are protected and that outbreaks are minimized. The scientific evidence overwhelmingly supports the use of vaccines as the best method for preventing infectious diseases and protecting public health.

Myth #4: Vaccines Are Unnecessary in a Modern World

In the modern age, with advancements in healthcare, sanitation, and technology, some people argue that vaccines are unnecessary. The belief is that modern medicine, better hygiene, and improved living conditions have rendered vaccines obsolete. Proponents of this myth often point to the dramatic decline in infectious diseases due to these factors and claim that vaccines are no longer needed. However, this myth ignores several important points about how diseases can still pose a threat in today's world and the irreplaceable role that vaccines play in preventing them.

The Origin of the Myth

The myth that vaccines are unnecessary in the modern world likely arises from the perception that diseases such as polio, smallpox, and measles are no longer major public health threats. While it's true that many vaccine-preventable diseases are much less common than they used to be, the reality is that they have not been eradicated completely. The success of vaccines in reducing the incidence of infectious diseases has created a false sense of security for some, leading them to believe that these diseases are a thing of the past.

Why Vaccines Are Still Crucial

1. **The Return of Preventable Diseases**:
    o One of the most significant reasons vaccines remain necessary, even in a modern world, is the potential for vaccine-preventable diseases to return if vaccination rates decline. Diseases like measles, whooping cough, and even polio have made comebacks in recent years, largely due to drops in vaccination rates. These diseases can spread quickly, especially when vaccination coverage falls below a certain threshold.

    o For example, in the United States and other developed countries, the resurgence of measles outbreaks in recent years is a direct result of declining vaccination rates and misinformation about vaccine safety. Without widespread vaccination, these diseases can quickly spread and cause significant harm to vulnerable populations, including infants, the elderly, and those with compromised immune systems.

2. **Global Travel and Disease Spread**:

    o   In today's interconnected world, people travel more than ever before, and infectious diseases can spread rapidly across borders. A person infected with a disease in one part of the world can unknowingly carry it to another country, where it can infect individuals who have not been vaccinated.

    o   Vaccines act as a defense against this global spread of disease. Even in countries with advanced healthcare systems, the risks posed by international travel make vaccination an essential tool for preventing outbreaks. For example, cases of diseases like tuberculosis, yellow fever, and Zika virus have been linked to global travel, and vaccines are often the only effective way to control their spread.

3. **New and Emerging Infectious Diseases**:

    o   Modern medicine and technology have helped us understand infectious diseases better, but new pathogens are still emerging. Diseases like COVID-19, H1N1 (swine flu), and Ebola have proven that we are still vulnerable to new and evolving infectious threats. Vaccines have played a critical role in controlling these outbreaks and preventing widespread illness.

○ Vaccination is a critical tool in the fight against emerging diseases. In the case of COVID-19, for example, the rapid development of vaccines helped slow the spread of the virus, reduce the severity of illness, and save millions of lives worldwide. Without vaccines, controlling the spread of such diseases would be much more difficult, if not impossible.

4. **Herd Immunity and Protection of Vulnerable Populations**:

○ Vaccines not only protect the individual receiving them but also help protect others through herd immunity. When a large portion of the population is vaccinated, it reduces the overall spread of disease, helping protect those who cannot be vaccinated, such as infants too young to receive certain vaccines, individuals with allergies or medical conditions, and those with weakened immune systems.

- In a modern world, where people are living longer and more individuals have chronic health conditions or are immunocompromised, herd immunity is crucial in preventing outbreaks and protecting the most vulnerable members of society.

5. **Vaccines Prevent More Than Just Infections**:

  - Vaccines do more than prevent the immediate threat of infectious diseases. Some vaccines protect against conditions that can cause long-term harm, including certain cancers. For example, the human papillomavirus (HPV) vaccine prevents infections that can lead to cervical, throat, and other cancers. The hepatitis B vaccine can prevent liver cancer. These vaccines represent not only an advancement in infectious disease prevention but also a critical step forward in cancer prevention.

  - Vaccines help reduce the overall burden of disease in society by preventing both immediate illness and long-term health consequences.

6. **The Role of Vaccines in Public Health Eradication Efforts**:

  - Some diseases, such as smallpox, have been eradicated thanks to global vaccination efforts. Polio is on the brink of eradication due to a concerted worldwide vaccination campaign. Without vaccines, these diseases would still be a global threat, causing millions of deaths and disabilities every year.

o The success of vaccination programs in eradicating or significantly reducing the prevalence of diseases like smallpox and polio demonstrates the immense value of vaccines in the modern world. While some may believe vaccines are no longer necessary, the reality is that without them, these diseases would return, and the progress made in public health could be reversed.

7. **Antibiotic Resistance and the Need for Prevention:**

o In a world where antibiotic resistance is becoming an increasing concern, vaccines play an even more important role in preventing diseases that would otherwise require antibiotic treatment. Preventing infections through vaccination can reduce the use of antibiotics and help mitigate the rise of antibiotic-resistant bacteria, which are a significant public health threat.

The Impact of Vaccine Hesitancy

Vaccine hesitancy, often fueled by misinformation, has led to a decline in vaccination rates in certain regions, putting public health at risk. The idea that vaccines are unnecessary in the modern world contributes to this hesitancy. When people believe that vaccines are no longer needed or that diseases no longer pose a serious threat, they may choose not to vaccinate themselves or their children, increasing the risk of outbreaks and putting vulnerable populations at greater risk.

Conclusion

Vaccines are more important than ever in the modern world. While advancements in healthcare and living conditions have certainly contributed to a decrease in the burden of infectious diseases, they have not made vaccines unnecessary. The reality is that without vaccines, we would still face the threat of preventable diseases, and the progress made in public health could be undone. Vaccines are essential not only for protecting individuals but also for safeguarding entire communities and preventing the resurgence of dangerous diseases. In a globalized world with emerging threats, vaccines remain one of the most effective tools we have to maintain public health and prevent widespread illness.

Debunking Common Vaccine Myths with Science

The spread of misinformation and misunderstandings about vaccines has contributed to vaccine hesitancy and the perpetuation of myths about their safety and efficacy. This section addresses and debunks some of the most common myths surrounding vaccines, providing scientific evidence to clarify misconceptions and offer a deeper understanding of the facts.

Myth #1: Vaccines Cause Autism

One of the most persistent and harmful myths is the claim that vaccines, particularly the MMR (measles, mumps, and rubella) vaccine, cause autism. This myth originated from a 1998 study by Andrew Wakefield, which was later discredited and retracted due to ethical concerns and falsified data. Despite this, the myth continues to circulate, fueled by misinformation.

Scientific Evidence: Numerous large-scale studies have thoroughly examined the potential link between vaccines and autism. A 2019 review involving over 650,000 children found no increased risk of autism associated with the MMR vaccine. The U.S. Centers for Disease Control and Prevention (CDC), World Health Organization (WHO), and other leading health organizations consistently affirm that vaccines do not cause autism. The real cause of autism is still not fully understood, but it is believed to be related to genetic factors and early brain development, not vaccines.

Myth #2: Vaccines Overwhelm the Immune System

Another myth is that vaccines overload the immune system by introducing too many antigens, especially when multiple vaccines are given in one visit. This myth suggests that the body can't handle so many vaccines at once and that this could weaken the immune system or lead to long-term health issues.

Scientific Evidence: The human immune system is capable of handling much more than the small number of antigens introduced by vaccines. In fact, we are constantly exposed to millions of antigens from everyday encounters with bacteria, viruses, and other microorganisms. The vaccines given in combination today use only a fraction of the immune system's potential to respond, and they do so in a controlled way. Research shows that the immune system can respond effectively to the many vaccines given during childhood without any adverse effects on immune function.

Myth #3: Natural Immunity Is Better Than Vaccine-Induced Immunity

Some people believe that natural immunity, which occurs when a person contracts and recovers from an infection, is superior to vaccine-induced immunity. While natural immunity can provide protection, this myth ignores the risks involved in allowing diseases to run their course, especially when vaccines are available.

Scientific Evidence: Natural immunity may provide long-lasting protection, but it comes at a significant risk. Diseases like measles, mumps, and chickenpox can cause serious complications, including hospitalization, brain damage, and death. Vaccines offer a safer alternative by providing immunity without exposing individuals to the dangers of the actual disease. For instance, the MMR vaccine not only protects against measles, mumps, and rubella but does so without the risk of severe complications, which can be life-threatening in some cases. Additionally, vaccines can provide more reliable immunity, especially against diseases that have a high risk of causing serious illness in vulnerable populations.

Myth #4: Vaccines Are Unnecessary in a Modern World

As discussed earlier, some people argue that vaccines are no longer necessary due to the improvement of public health, sanitation, and medical care. They believe that diseases like measles and polio are a thing of the past and that we no longer need vaccines to protect against these illnesses.

Scientific Evidence: While modern healthcare has undoubtedly reduced the burden of many infectious diseases, vaccines remain a critical tool in preventing outbreaks. Diseases like measles, polio, and whooping cough are still present in many parts of the world and can easily spread, especially if vaccination rates drop. The resurgence of diseases previously thought to be eradicated, such as measles in the U.S. and other developed countries, underscores the continuing importance of vaccination. Vaccines also protect not only individuals but also communities, especially those who cannot be vaccinated due to medical reasons (e.g., infants, immunocompromised individuals).

Myth #5: Vaccines Contain Harmful Ingredients

A common myth is that vaccines contain dangerous levels of harmful ingredients such as mercury, formaldehyde, or aluminum. These substances are often cited as being toxic, leading some to believe that vaccines are unsafe.

Scientific Evidence: While it's true that some vaccines contain trace amounts of ingredients like aluminum salts (used to enhance the immune response) or formaldehyde (used in vaccine production to inactivate viruses), these substances are present in such small quantities that they pose no harm. In fact, the amount of aluminum found in vaccines is much smaller than what a person encounters in daily life through food, water, and air. The mercury used in vaccines (thimerosal) has been removed from most childhood vaccines, except for some multi-dose flu vaccines. Even when thimerosal was used, it was in a concentration that was not harmful. Extensive research and testing by health authorities such as the U.S. Food and Drug Administration (FDA) and the CDC ensure that vaccine ingredients are safe and effective in the doses used.

Myth #6: Vaccines Cause Sudden Infant Death Syndrome (SIDS)

Another myth is that vaccines are a leading cause of Sudden Infant Death Syndrome (SIDS). This misconception is often based on the fact that SIDS occurs in infants, typically between 2 and 4 months of age, which is also when infants receive several routine vaccines.

Scientific Evidence: There is no scientific evidence linking vaccines to SIDS. Numerous studies have examined this claim, and none have found a connection between vaccines and SIDS. In fact, some studies suggest that vaccination may actually lower the risk of SIDS. Vaccines save lives by preventing serious infections in infants and young children, and their safety is well established through decades of research and monitoring.

Myth #7: Vaccines Are Only Necessary for Children

While vaccines are essential for children, many believe that adults no longer need vaccinations after childhood. This myth neglects the fact that immunity can wane over time, and that some vaccines need to be updated to continue providing protection.

Scientific Evidence: Adults also require vaccines to maintain immunity against diseases like tetanus, diphtheria, pertussis (whooping cough), and shingles. For example, the Tdap booster is recommended for adults to maintain protection against tetanus, diphtheria, and pertussis. Influenza and pneumonia vaccines are also important for older adults, as they are at higher risk for complications from these diseases. The HPV vaccine, which prevents several cancers, is recommended for adults up to age 45. Vaccines are essential throughout life to ensure continued protection against infectious diseases.

Conclusion: The Power of Science in Vaccine Understanding

Debunking these common vaccine myths with science is essential in clearing the air around vaccination. The myths often stem from misunderstandings or deliberate misinformation, but the evidence is clear: vaccines are safe, effective, and necessary to protect both individual and public health. As we move forward, it is crucial to continue to rely on scientific research, expert recommendations, and evidence-based data to guide vaccine policy and personal health decisions.

Chapter 5: Herd Immunity: The Cornerstone of Public Health

Herd immunity, also known as community immunity, is a concept in public health that describes how a disease is unable to spread within a population when a sufficient portion of that population becomes immune to it. This immunity can be achieved through vaccination or prior infection. In essence, when most people are immune, the spread of infectious diseases slows or stops, which helps protect individuals who are not immune—either because they are too young, have medical conditions preventing vaccination, or cannot be vaccinated for other reasons.

How Does Herd Immunity Work?

The primary mechanism behind herd immunity is reducing the overall spread of an infectious disease. When a large percentage of people are immune to a disease, it reduces the number of individuals who can carry and transmit the pathogen. This makes it harder for the disease to find vulnerable individuals to infect, thereby lowering the chance of an outbreak.

Here's a closer look at the processes that make herd immunity work:

1. **Immunity Reduces Transmission**: Immune individuals are less likely to get infected by the disease, and therefore, they are less likely to spread it. In turn, the fewer people who are capable of transmitting the disease, the slower the disease spreads.

2. **Protection for Vulnerable Individuals**: Herd immunity is especially important for people who cannot be vaccinated—such as infants, elderly individuals, pregnant women, and those with weakened immune systems due to diseases like cancer. These individuals rely on the immunity of those around them to protect them from exposure to diseases that they are particularly vulnerable to.

3. **Threshold of Immunity**: For herd immunity to be effective, a certain percentage of the population must be immune. This percentage depends on the specific disease and how contagious it is. For example, diseases like measles, which are highly contagious, require about 95% of the population to be immune to prevent widespread transmission. For less contagious diseases, a lower percentage might suffice.

The Role of Vaccination in Achieving Herd Immunity

Vaccination is the most effective way to build herd immunity. Vaccines help individuals develop immunity without having to experience the illness itself. By ensuring a high percentage of people are vaccinated, public health authorities can control the spread of diseases and protect vulnerable populations.

In some cases, herd immunity has been achieved for certain diseases through widespread vaccination campaigns. For example:

- **Smallpox**: Smallpox was eradicated globally in 1980 due to widespread vaccination efforts that created herd immunity.

- **Polio**: Through vaccination, polio has been largely eradicated in many parts of the world, though some countries still face challenges.

What Happens If Herd Immunity Is Not Achieved?

If vaccination rates decrease or if there is vaccine hesitancy, herd immunity becomes more difficult to maintain, and diseases can resurge. For example, recent outbreaks of measles in certain areas can be attributed to a decline in vaccination rates, resulting in the breakdown of herd immunity.

Without herd immunity, individuals who are vulnerable to diseases—such as newborns, the elderly, or those with compromised immune systems—are at a much higher risk of contracting serious illnesses. This can lead to higher hospitalization rates, increased mortality, and the burden of disease on the healthcare system.

The Threshold for Herd Immunity

The threshold for achieving herd immunity depends on how contagious the disease is. This is measured using the **basic reproduction number (R0)**, which refers to the average number of people who will become infected from one person with the disease. The higher the R0, the more individuals need to be immune to stop the spread of the disease.

For example:

- **Measles**: The R0 for measles is 12 to 18, meaning that 95% of the population needs to be immune to stop its spread.

- **Polio**: The R0 for polio is lower, around 5 to 7, so 80-85% of the population needs to be immune.

- **Influenza**: The R0 for influenza is around 1.3 to 2, meaning that herd immunity can be achieved with a vaccination rate of around 60-80%.

Factors That Affect Herd Immunity

Several factors can influence how easily herd immunity can be achieved and maintained:

- **Vaccine Efficacy**: The effectiveness of a vaccine determines how many people need to be vaccinated to achieve herd immunity. If a vaccine is highly effective, fewer people need to be vaccinated.

- **Population Density**: In densely populated areas, the risk of transmission is higher, so higher vaccination rates are needed to create herd immunity.

- **Vaccine Hesitancy**: Public reluctance or refusal to vaccinate can decrease vaccination coverage, weakening herd immunity and making outbreaks more likely.

- **Access to Vaccines**: For herd immunity to be achieved on a broad scale, vaccines must be accessible to all populations, including those in remote or underserved areas.

Why Herd Immunity Matters

Herd immunity is a critical tool for preventing the spread of infectious diseases, especially for those who are most vulnerable. Achieving herd immunity can:

- **Protect Those Who Can't Be Vaccinated**: It provides indirect protection to individuals who cannot receive vaccines due to medical reasons.

- **Prevent Disease Outbreaks**: It helps keep disease outbreaks at bay, reducing the incidence of illness, hospitalization, and death.

- **Protect Public Health**: It lowers the overall burden on healthcare systems, preventing hospitals from being overwhelmed during disease outbreaks.

In conclusion, herd immunity is a vital mechanism in the fight against infectious diseases. Achieving and maintaining herd immunity through widespread vaccination not only protects individuals but also strengthens public health systems by preventing the spread of dangerous diseases.

Can Vaccines Achieve Herd Immunity?

Yes, vaccines can and have achieved herd immunity for various infectious diseases. Vaccination is the most effective method to build immunity within a population and prevent the spread of disease. The goal of herd immunity through vaccination is to protect individuals who cannot be vaccinated or are at higher risk of severe outcomes by reducing the overall circulation of the disease. Here's how vaccines contribute to achieving herd immunity and why they are essential for public health:

How Vaccines Achieve Herd Immunity

Vaccination works by introducing a harmless component of a pathogen (such as a weakened or inactivated virus, or a piece of the pathogen like a protein) to stimulate the immune system. This allows the body to recognize and fight the pathogen if it encounters it in the future, without causing illness. When enough people are vaccinated, the following happens:

1. **Reduction in Disease Transmission**: As more individuals become immune (either from vaccination or previous infection), fewer people are susceptible to the disease. This makes it harder for the disease to spread because there are fewer potential hosts for the pathogen to infect.

2. **Protecting Vulnerable Populations**: Some individuals cannot receive vaccines due to medical conditions, age, or other reasons (such as allergies or compromised immune systems). These individuals rely on the immunity of the general population to reduce the likelihood of exposure to infectious diseases. When herd immunity is achieved, the disease has fewer opportunities to spread to these vulnerable groups.

3. **Breaking the Chain of Transmission**: In a population where most people are immune, the pathogen struggles to find enough susceptible hosts to sustain transmission. Even if a small proportion of people remain susceptible, the disease's ability to spread is drastically reduced.

Examples of Vaccines That Have Achieved Herd Immunity

There are numerous examples of vaccines achieving herd immunity and leading to the control or even eradication of diseases:

1. **Measles**: Measles is a highly contagious disease with an R0 (basic reproduction number) of 12 to 18. This means that 95% of the population needs to be immune to stop the disease from spreading. Through widespread vaccination, many countries have been able to achieve herd immunity for measles, drastically reducing its incidence. However, recent declines in vaccination rates in some areas have led to

outbreaks, illustrating the importance of maintaining high vaccination coverage.

2. **Polio**: Polio is another example where vaccination has led to herd immunity and, in many parts of the world, near eradication. By vaccinating large populations, the spread of polio has been reduced so significantly that the disease is no longer endemic in most countries. The Global Polio Eradication Initiative has brought the world to the brink of eradicating polio entirely, though challenges remain in certain regions.

3. **Influenza**: Although influenza vaccines are not as effective in achieving herd immunity as vaccines for diseases like measles, widespread vaccination can still reduce the severity and spread of the disease. In flu seasons with high vaccination coverage, the overall burden of flu-related illness is significantly reduced.

4. **COVID-19**: The COVID-19 pandemic has shown how vaccines can contribute to achieving herd immunity. Although COVID-19 vaccines have not fully eradicated the virus, they have played a crucial role in reducing transmission and preventing severe illness and death. With enough individuals vaccinated, the virus's ability to spread in the community decreases, helping to protect vulnerable populations.

Factors Affecting Vaccine-Induced Herd Immunity

Achieving herd immunity through vaccines depends on several factors:

1. **Vaccine Efficacy**: The effectiveness of a vaccine in preventing disease is crucial. If a vaccine does not provide strong protection, it is less likely to contribute to herd immunity. Some vaccines, like the measles vaccine, are highly effective at preventing disease, while others may have lower efficacy, which affects how much of the population needs to be vaccinated.

2. **Vaccine Coverage**: For herd immunity to be achieved, a sufficient percentage of the population must be vaccinated. This threshold depends on the contagiousness of the disease (its R0). For highly contagious diseases like measles, this can be as high as 95%. If vaccination rates drop, the likelihood of outbreaks increases, and herd immunity becomes harder to maintain.

3. **Vaccine Hesitancy**: Vaccine hesitancy, or the refusal to vaccinate despite the availability of vaccines, is a significant challenge to achieving herd immunity. Misinformation and distrust in vaccines can reduce vaccination rates, making it difficult to reach the levels required for herd immunity.

4. **Global Vaccination Efforts**: Achieving herd immunity is not just about vaccination within a single country; it requires global efforts. Diseases like polio, for example, can spread across borders, so vaccination must be widespread to prevent global transmission.

5. **Disease Mutations**: Some pathogens, like the flu and COVID-19, can mutate, which can affect the ability of vaccines to maintain their efficacy over time. For example, new variants of a virus may evade immunity, requiring updated vaccines and booster doses to maintain herd immunity.

6. **Population Mobility**: Movement of people across regions can affect herd immunity. Travelers from areas with lower vaccination rates can introduce infectious diseases into populations that have achieved herd immunity, leading to potential outbreaks if vaccination rates are not maintained.

Challenges to Achieving Herd Immunity with Vaccines

While vaccines can achieve herd immunity, there are challenges that must be overcome to ensure success:

- **Vaccine Access**: In many parts of the world, access to vaccines is limited due to economic, geographic, or political factors. Widespread vaccination requires global efforts to ensure vaccines are available to everyone, including those in low-income countries.

- **Vaccine Distribution**: Even when vaccines are available, the logistics of distributing them to all populations, particularly in remote areas, can be challenging. Cold chain requirements, transportation, and healthcare infrastructure all play a role in how effectively vaccines can be delivered.

- **Vaccine Uptake**: The success of vaccination programs depends on high levels of acceptance and uptake. Public education, combating misinformation, and building trust in healthcare systems are essential to achieving and maintaining herd immunity.

Conclusion

Vaccines are a powerful tool in achieving herd immunity, and they have already successfully controlled or eradicated numerous diseases. By vaccinating large portions of the population, we can reduce disease transmission, protect vulnerable individuals, and ultimately improve public health. However, achieving herd immunity requires ongoing efforts to ensure high vaccination rates, address vaccine hesitancy, and improve access to vaccines globally. While vaccines are not a panacea, they are one of the most effective public health measures available to prevent the spread of infectious diseases and protect individuals and communities from harm.

The Challenges of Herd Immunity in a Diverse Population

Achieving herd immunity through vaccination is a crucial goal in public health, but it comes with unique challenges in diverse and heterogeneous populations. Differences in access to healthcare, varying levels of trust in medical systems, cultural beliefs, socioeconomic factors, and geographic mobility all contribute to the complexity of establishing herd immunity across a population. This section explores these challenges and the ways they impact efforts to reach and maintain sufficient immunity levels to control or eradicate infectious diseases.

1. Variability in Vaccine Access

Access to vaccines is not uniform across populations, often affected by geographic, economic, and political factors. In underserved areas, healthcare infrastructure may be lacking, making it difficult to distribute vaccines effectively. Additionally, marginalized communities may face barriers to healthcare services, including lack of insurance, transportation, and education about vaccine availability. To achieve herd immunity, addressing these disparities and ensuring equitable access to vaccines is essential.

2. Vaccine Hesitancy and Cultural Beliefs

Vaccine hesitancy, influenced by personal beliefs, cultural practices, and misinformation, is a significant barrier to achieving herd immunity. Some communities may have historical mistrust of medical institutions, especially if they have experienced discrimination or unethical medical practices in the past. Cultural beliefs about health and medicine may also impact individuals' willingness to vaccinate. Public health initiatives must work to build trust, engage with community leaders, and provide culturally sensitive information to address these concerns and encourage vaccination.

3. Socioeconomic Inequities and Health Disparities

Socioeconomic factors, such as income, education level, and living conditions, can influence vaccination rates and, by extension, herd immunity. Lower-income communities may have limited healthcare access, and individuals with lower education levels may be less aware of the benefits and availability of vaccines. Furthermore, people living in crowded or inadequate housing may be at higher risk for infectious diseases but face greater barriers to vaccination. Policies aimed at reducing these disparities are critical for achieving herd immunity on a broad scale.

4. Geographic Mobility and Transient Populations

The movement of people within and across borders presents challenges to maintaining herd immunity. Urban centers, which often have more mobile populations, can experience fluctuations in immunity levels due to transient groups, such as migrants, travelers, and seasonal workers. These populations may have varying levels of vaccine coverage, and they can unintentionally introduce infectious diseases to regions where immunity is high, leading to outbreaks. Coordinating vaccination efforts across regions and countries is essential to address this issue and to prevent the spread of diseases.

5. Varying Immune Responses and Health Conditions

Individual differences in immune responses can affect the effectiveness of vaccines and the overall level of immunity within a population. Factors such as age, underlying health conditions, and immunocompromised status can impact how well a vaccine works for certain individuals. For example, elderly adults or people with certain chronic diseases may not develop as strong an immune response to vaccines as healthy, younger individuals. This makes it even more crucial to ensure high vaccination rates among the general population to protect those who may not have full immunity.

6. Misinformation and Social Media Influence

In today's digital age, misinformation about vaccines spreads rapidly, often fueled by social media. Conspiracy theories and misleading information can quickly undermine public trust and lead to reduced vaccination rates, even in communities with high vaccine access. Combating misinformation requires proactive public health communication strategies, including the involvement of trusted community figures and evidence-based messaging to counteract myths and provide accurate information.

7. Political and Policy Barriers

In some regions, political and policy-related factors can hinder vaccination campaigns. Differences in health policy between local, state, and national governments can result in inconsistent vaccine distribution and promotion strategies. Political polarization around public health measures may also lead to resistance to vaccination campaigns, especially if they are perceived as infringing on personal freedom. Coordinating policy efforts across political divides is critical for achieving herd immunity in a diverse population.

8. Logistic and Supply Chain Challenges

Logistical challenges, such as the need for cold storage, transportation, and adequate staffing, complicate vaccine distribution, particularly in remote or rural areas. Supply chain issues can result in vaccine shortages, delaying immunization efforts and compromising herd immunity. Ensuring a robust and resilient supply chain, along with investing in healthcare infrastructure, is essential to meet the needs of diverse populations and maintain consistent vaccination coverage.

9. Balancing Public Health with Individual Rights

The concept of herd immunity often requires high vaccination rates, which may lead to public health mandates, such as mandatory vaccination for certain groups (e.g., healthcare workers or students). However, balancing public health needs with respect for individual autonomy and freedom can be challenging. Public health policies must carefully navigate this balance, aiming to protect communities while considering individual rights and cultural sensitivities.

10. Addressing Global Disparities for Worldwide Herd Immunity

Global connectivity means that achieving herd immunity in one country is not sufficient if other regions remain unvaccinated. Infectious diseases do not respect borders, and outbreaks in one area can spread rapidly to others. International collaboration is essential for achieving herd immunity worldwide, especially in low-resource settings where vaccination rates may be lower. Supporting global vaccination efforts, such as those led by organizations like the World Health Organization and Gavi, the Vaccine Alliance, can help address this challenge.

These diverse challenges highlight the complexities of achieving herd immunity in a globalized and heterogeneous world. Success requires a multifaceted approach that includes improving vaccine accessibility, building public trust, addressing misinformation, and fostering collaboration across communities and governments. While achieving herd immunity is a formidable goal, it remains a vital strategy in reducing the burden of infectious diseases and promoting public health for all.

The Consequences of Failing to Achieve Herd Immunity

When herd immunity is not achieved, a population faces several potential risks and consequences. Herd immunity acts as a protective barrier, shielding those who cannot be vaccinated or those who are more vulnerable to disease. Failing to reach this level of immunity compromises not only individual health but also community and global health stability. This section explores the far-reaching implications of insufficient herd immunity and how it can lead to increased disease outbreaks, strain on healthcare systems, economic impacts, and greater public health challenges.

1. Increased Outbreaks and Epidemics

Without sufficient herd immunity, infectious diseases can spread rapidly through communities, leading to frequent outbreaks. These outbreaks can quickly escalate to epidemics, especially in densely populated areas where people interact closely. Diseases like measles, which are highly contagious, can have devastating impacts when a population's immunity level drops below the threshold needed to prevent transmission. Increased outbreaks mean a greater number of people falling ill, more hospitalizations, and higher death rates, especially among vulnerable populations.

2. Higher Morbidity and Mortality Rates

When infectious diseases circulate freely due to low immunity, morbidity (the rate of disease) and mortality (the rate of death) increase. Diseases like influenza, measles, and whooping cough can be particularly severe for infants, the elderly, and immunocompromised individuals. For some diseases, especially those without effective treatments, failing to reach herd immunity can result in prolonged illnesses, serious complications, and even fatalities, particularly among those who rely on community immunity for protection.

3. Overburdened Healthcare Systems

Frequent disease outbreaks lead to a higher demand for healthcare services, placing a significant strain on hospitals, clinics, and healthcare workers. During widespread outbreaks, healthcare systems may become overwhelmed, leading to bed shortages, delays in treatment, and limited access to critical care. This strain affects not only those with the disease but also patients seeking care for other medical needs, as resources are diverted to handle outbreaks. The consequences include longer wait times, compromised care quality, and even burnout among healthcare professionals.

4. Economic Consequences

Widespread disease outbreaks have considerable economic costs, impacting both individuals and the broader economy. These costs arise from increased healthcare expenses, lost productivity, workplace absences, and disruptions to business operations. Additionally, governments may need to allocate extra resources to outbreak response efforts, which can strain budgets and divert funds from other essential services. Travel restrictions, school closures, and quarantine measures during severe outbreaks further contribute to economic losses, affecting sectors like tourism, retail, and education.

5. Threats to Vulnerable Populations

Certain individuals depend heavily on herd immunity for protection, including newborns, the elderly, pregnant women, and people with compromised immune systems. When a community falls short of herd immunity, these vulnerable groups face a higher risk of infection. For some, vaccination is either less effective or not possible, making them especially reliant on community protection. Failing to achieve herd immunity puts their health and safety at considerable risk, potentially leading to severe health outcomes or loss of life.

6. Re-emergence of Previously Controlled Diseases

Insufficient vaccination coverage can lead to the re-emergence of diseases that were previously under control or even eradicated in certain areas. Examples include measles and mumps, which have resurged in regions where vaccine coverage declined. When immunity levels drop, diseases that were nearly eliminated can make a comeback, undoing decades of public health progress and requiring renewed efforts to contain outbreaks. This backslide in disease control highlights the critical importance of maintaining high vaccination rates.

7. Weakened Public Confidence in Health Measures

When outbreaks occur due to insufficient herd immunity, public trust in health measures and vaccination programs can weaken. Some individuals may misinterpret rising case numbers as evidence that vaccines are ineffective, leading to further vaccine hesitancy. Public confidence is crucial for the success of health campaigns; if people lose trust in vaccines, it becomes even more challenging to achieve herd immunity and protect public health.

8. Increased Healthcare Costs for Individuals and Society

Without herd immunity, individuals and communities face higher healthcare costs, both direct and indirect. Direct costs include medical expenses for treating disease-related complications, while indirect costs encompass lost workdays, caregiver expenses, and long-term health impacts. When disease rates increase, healthcare spending rises accordingly, burdening not only individuals but also public health resources. Taxpayer-funded healthcare systems bear the additional cost of managing preventable diseases, diverting funds from other health initiatives.

9. Long-term Health Complications

Failing to control infectious diseases through herd immunity can lead to long-term health complications in those affected by severe cases. Diseases such as measles, polio, and whooping cough can cause chronic health issues or permanent disability, impacting a person's quality of life for years to come. Complications like encephalitis, organ damage, or respiratory issues add a lifelong health burden on survivors and require ongoing medical attention and support.

10. Global Health Risks

In an interconnected world, infectious diseases can easily cross borders. A lack of herd immunity in one region can create a domino effect, spreading disease to other areas, including those with high immunity levels. This can lead to outbreaks in populations that may otherwise be protected, posing a risk to global health. Countries with insufficient herd immunity act as reservoirs for infectious agents, increasing the likelihood of mutation and the emergence of new, potentially more virulent strains that can spread globally.

The consequences of failing to achieve herd immunity extend far beyond individual illness, affecting entire communities, economies, and public health systems. Maintaining high vaccination rates and striving for herd immunity are crucial steps in protecting both current and future generations from the potentially severe impacts of preventable infectious diseases.

Chapter 6: Historical Perspectives: Vaccines and the Decline of Infectious Diseases

The Role of Vaccines in Eradicating Diseases

This section focuses on how vaccines have played a pivotal role in the eradication and near-elimination of some of the world's most devastating infectious diseases. By highlighting success stories and ongoing efforts, readers can gain insight into the powerful impact vaccines have had on global health and the challenges still faced in the fight against infectious diseases.

---

1. The Historical Significance of Smallpox Eradication

- **A Global Effort to Eliminate Smallpox**: The unprecedented, coordinated international campaign led by the World Health Organization.

- **Strategies for Success**: The use of ring vaccination, tracking and isolation, and community involvement.

- **Lessons Learned from Smallpox**: How the eradication of smallpox in 1980 provided a blueprint for addressing other infectious diseases.

2. Polio Eradication: A Work in Progress

- **The Devastation of Polio Epidemics**: Understanding the impact of polio outbreaks and the motivation behind global eradication efforts.

- **The Success of the Polio Vaccine**: How the introduction of the inactivated (IPV) and oral (OPV) polio vaccines dramatically reduced cases worldwide.

- **Challenges to Complete Eradication**: The current obstacles, such as vaccine-resistant strains, political barriers, and maintaining high immunization rates in vulnerable regions.

3. Measles and Rubella: The Path to Elimination

- **Vaccination as a Tool to Control and Prevent Outbreaks**: The effectiveness of the MMR (measles, mumps, and rubella) vaccine in reducing disease spread.

- **Eradication Efforts and Setbacks**: The goal of eliminating measles and rubella, hindered by vaccine hesitancy and gaps in vaccination coverage.

- **The Importance of Global Immunization Campaigns**: How coordinated efforts can bring these diseases closer to eradication.

4. Challenges in Eradicating Other Vaccine-Preventable Diseases

- **Hepatitis B and C**: The progress and challenges in controlling and eliminating chronic infections through vaccination.

- **Human Papillomavirus (HPV)**: How HPV vaccination campaigns aim to reduce and potentially eliminate HPV-related cancers.

- **Emerging Threats and Evolving Vaccination Needs**: The role of vaccines in combating diseases like malaria, tuberculosis, and HIV, and the scientific hurdles in developing effective vaccines.

5. The Impact of Vaccine Hesitancy on Eradication Efforts

- **Understanding Vaccine Hesitancy**: Factors that contribute to resistance to vaccination and their impact on disease control.

- **Outbreaks in Unvaccinated Populations**: How vaccine hesitancy has led to resurgences of diseases previously controlled by vaccines.

- **Strategies for Overcoming Hesitancy**: Public health approaches to rebuilding trust and encouraging widespread vaccine acceptance.

6. Future Directions for Vaccine-Driven Disease Eradication

- **Advances in Vaccine Technology**: The role of mRNA and vector-based vaccines in speeding up disease control efforts.

- **The Role of International Collaboration**: How countries and organizations are working together to achieve eradication goals.

- **Looking Ahead**: Potential targets for eradication and the importance of maintaining high vaccination rates for ongoing public health.

By examining the history and current status of vaccine-driven disease eradication, this section underscores the immense role that vaccines have played—and continue to play—in reducing the global burden of infectious diseases. The triumphs, challenges, and future possibilities reflect both the power and complexity of using vaccination as a tool to protect public health worldwide.

The Decline of Smallpox, Polio, and Other Vaccine-Preventable Diseases

This section delves into the remarkable public health achievements resulting from vaccination efforts that have led to the decline of once-devastating diseases, such as smallpox and polio. It also explores how vaccines have transformed the landscape of infectious disease prevention by targeting other serious illnesses, providing historical and scientific context to highlight the profound impact of immunization on global health.

---

1. Smallpox: The First Vaccine Success Story

- **The Severity of Smallpox Before Vaccination**: How smallpox plagued populations with high mortality and widespread suffering.

- **Edward Jenner and the First Vaccine**: The development of the first smallpox vaccine in the late 18th century and the beginning of modern immunology.

- **The Global Eradication Campaign**: Key milestones and the strategies that led to the official eradication of smallpox in 1980, a historic achievement in global health.

2. Polio: Near Eradication and Continued Efforts

- **The Toll of Polio Epidemics**: The crippling impact of polio before the introduction of vaccines and the motivation to eradicate it.

- **Development of the Polio Vaccines**: The creation of the inactivated (IPV) and oral (OPV) polio vaccines, and their role in dramatically reducing cases worldwide.

- **Challenges to Complete Eradication**: Ongoing obstacles, including outbreaks in unvaccinated areas, vaccine-derived poliovirus, and logistical hurdles in high-risk regions.

3. Measles, Mumps, and Rubella: Vaccination's Role in Controlling Outbreaks

- **The Introduction of the MMR Vaccine**: How the measles, mumps, and rubella (MMR) vaccine helped significantly reduce the incidence of these contagious diseases.

- **The Impact of Vaccination Campaigns**: How widespread MMR vaccination has limited outbreaks and prevented severe complications from these diseases.

- **Resurgence Concerns Due to Vaccine Hesitancy**: The role of declining vaccination rates in the resurgence of measles and the importance of maintaining high coverage.

4. Haemophilus Influenzae Type B (Hib): A Triumph Against Childhood Meningitis

- **The Dangers of Hib Prior to Vaccination**: The high risk of Hib infection, especially in young children, and its association with meningitis and pneumonia.

- **Development of the Hib Vaccine**: How introducing the Hib vaccine led to a sharp decrease in Hib-related illnesses and deaths.

- **Long-Term Impact**: The continued success of Hib vaccination in nearly eradicating severe Hib infections in vaccinated populations.

5. Rotavirus: Reducing Childhood Diarrheal Deaths

- **The Global Burden of Rotavirus**: The impact of rotavirus as a leading cause of severe diarrhea and death in young children.

- **Introduction of the Rotavirus Vaccine**: How rotavirus vaccination programs have drastically reduced hospitalizations and fatalities in countries with high vaccination coverage.

- **Challenges in Low-Resource Settings**: Efforts to expand rotavirus vaccination in low- and middle-income countries to further reduce childhood mortality.

6. Tetanus, Diphtheria, and Pertussis (DTP): Protecting Against Severe Bacterial Infections

- **The Introduction of the DTP Vaccine**: How the DTP combination vaccine has helped protect millions from tetanus, diphtheria, and pertussis (whooping cough).

- **Maintaining Immunization Coverage**: The importance of continued DTP vaccination to prevent outbreaks of these life-threatening infections, especially in vulnerable populations.

- **The Impact on Global Health**: How DTP vaccination campaigns have contributed to a dramatic decline in morbidity and mortality associated with these diseases.

7. Hepatitis B: Preventing Chronic Liver Disease and Cancer

- **The Risks of Hepatitis B Infection**: The potential for chronic infection leading to liver disease and liver cancer.

- **Widespread Implementation of Hepatitis B Vaccination**: The global push to vaccinate infants against hepatitis B to prevent chronic infections from developing.

- **Progress Toward Elimination**: The significant reduction in hepatitis B prevalence in countries with high vaccination coverage and efforts to expand access in high-burden regions.

This chapter presents a clear picture of how vaccines have led to the dramatic decline of these once-prevalent diseases, highlighting both the successes and ongoing efforts required to protect public health. By understanding the historical impact of vaccination, readers gain insight into the power of immunization as a tool for preventing suffering and improving quality of life on a global scale.

Was Vaccination the Only Factor in Declining Disease Rates?

we explore whether vaccination alone was responsible for the significant decline in disease rates over the last century or if other factors also played important roles. While vaccines have had a profound impact on reducing cases of many infectious diseases, understanding the broader context provides a more comprehensive view of public health progress.

---

1. The Role of Improved Sanitation and Hygiene

- **Advances in Clean Water and Sewage Systems**: How access to clean drinking water and effective sewage disposal helped reduce diseases spread through contaminated water and poor sanitation, such as cholera and typhoid.

- **Personal Hygiene Practices**: Increased awareness and practice of handwashing, especially in medical settings, and how it contributed to lowering infection rates.

2. Nutritional Improvements and Disease Resistance

- **Better Diets, Stronger Immune Systems**: The link between improved nutrition and the body's ability to resist infections. Malnutrition weakens immunity, making individuals more susceptible to infections.

- **Impact on Childhood Mortality**: How improved infant and child nutrition helped reduce the mortality rates from infectious diseases, even before the widespread use of vaccines.

3. Medical Advancements and Supportive Treatments

- **Antibiotics and Antiviral Treatments**: The introduction of antibiotics helped manage bacterial infections that sometimes arose as secondary infections in diseases like measles, reducing overall mortality.

- **Development of Supportive Care**: Advances in hospital care, such as IV fluids and oxygen therapy, improved survival rates for those affected by infectious diseases.

4. Socioeconomic Development and Access to Healthcare

- **Higher Standards of Living**: How socioeconomic progress, such as improved housing, reduced overcrowding, and access to healthcare, lowered the spread of infectious diseases.

- **Expanded Access to Medical Services**: The role of regular medical check-ups, early diagnosis, and access to immunization programs in controlling disease spread.

5. Public Health Campaigns and Education

- **Education on Disease Prevention**: Public health campaigns promoting handwashing, breastfeeding, and preventive health behaviors that help reduce infection risk.

- **Global and National Health Initiatives**: The impact of organizations like the World Health Organization and CDC in implementing large-scale public health strategies, including vaccine promotion and disease surveillance.

While vaccination has been one of the most impactful tools in reducing infectious disease rates, this section highlights that it is part of a broader web of public health advancements. Together, these factors have created a more resilient and healthier society, showing that while vaccines are powerful, a comprehensive approach to health and wellness has been essential in achieving lasting disease reduction.

The Importance of Vaccination in Global Health

Vaccination has been recognized as one of the most powerful tools in modern medicine, with widespread benefits for individual health and public safety. In this section, we'll examine the critical role that vaccines play in global health, protecting communities from devastating outbreaks, and reducing the burden on healthcare systems worldwide.

---

1. Preventing the Spread of Infectious Diseases

- **Protection at the Population Level**: How vaccines help create herd immunity, which shields vulnerable populations who may be unable to receive certain vaccines due to age or health conditions.

- **Controlling Outbreaks and Epidemics**: The effectiveness of vaccination campaigns in halting the spread of diseases like measles, polio, and influenza and limiting the impact of outbreaks.

2. Reducing Mortality and Morbidity

- **Saving Millions of Lives Annually**: Statistics and examples of diseases like smallpox and polio where vaccines have significantly reduced or eradicated fatalities.

- **Decreasing Long-Term Health Complications**: How vaccines not only prevent death but also reduce the incidence of severe complications, such as paralysis from polio or liver cancer from hepatitis B.

3. Economic Benefits of Vaccination

- **Reducing Healthcare Costs**: By preventing disease, vaccines help reduce medical expenses associated with treatment, hospitalizations, and long-term care.

- **Improving Workforce Productivity**: Healthier populations lead to fewer sick days, enhanced productivity, and more stable economies, particularly in developing nations.

4. Vaccination's Role in Achieving Global Health Goals

- **Alignment with United Nations Sustainable Development Goals**: How vaccines contribute to global targets like reducing child mortality and combating infectious diseases in developing countries.

- **Impact on Vulnerable Populations**: The role of vaccines in protecting at-risk groups, such as infants, the elderly, and those in low-resource settings, from preventable diseases.

5. Vaccination as a Public Health Milestone

- **The Success Story of Smallpox Eradication**: The global effort that led to the complete eradication of smallpox, and how it serves as a model for future eradication campaigns.

- **Future Targets for Disease Eradication**: Ongoing initiatives aimed at eradicating diseases like polio and measles through comprehensive vaccination programs.

Vaccination remains an essential component of public health infrastructure, contributing to the well-being and stability of societies around the globe. This section underscores the profound impact that vaccines have on reducing suffering, supporting economic development, and building a healthier world for future generations.

Chapter 7: The Controversies and Ethical Questions Surrounding Vaccines

The Ethics of Mandating Vaccines

- **Public Health vs. Individual Autonomy**

    o Examining the core ethical tension: public health's responsibility to protect society versus respecting individuals' autonomy over their health choices.

    o Analyzing philosophical and ethical frameworks that advocate for both sides, including the principle of harm reduction versus personal liberty.

    o How mandates are justified in the context of highly contagious diseases versus less transmissible ones.

- **Historical Precedents for Vaccine Mandates**

    o A look at notable mandates throughout history, such as smallpox vaccination in the 19th century, and the public's varied reactions.

    o Successes and challenges in past vaccine mandates, including public resistance, enforcement issues, and the impact on disease control.

- Learning from past instances where mandates were imposed or rejected, including the role of public trust in compliance.

- **Legal Frameworks and Exemptions**

  - Understanding the legal underpinnings of mandates in different countries, such as U.S. states' power to mandate vaccines for school children and healthcare workers.

  - Detailed discussion of religious, medical, and personal belief exemptions, their origins, and the controversies surrounding them.

  - The balance between protecting public health and respecting individuals' rights under the law; examining court cases and landmark rulings related to vaccine mandates.

- **Informed Consent and Medical Autonomy**

  - Exploring the ethical principle of informed consent and how it applies to vaccine mandates, including information transparency and the right to refuse treatment.

  - The nuances of medical autonomy in the context of public health interventions, and where the line is drawn in cases where individual choices could impact community health.

- Examining whether mandates compromise informed consent, especially when exemptions are limited or difficult to obtain.

- **Impact on Vulnerable and Marginalized Populations**

  - Assessing how vaccine mandates affect populations with limited healthcare access, mistrust of medical institutions, or cultural hesitancy toward vaccines.

  - The disproportionate burden mandates may place on specific groups, and how policies can be designed to be more inclusive and equitable.

  - Exploring efforts to improve outreach and access to vaccination to avoid punitive measures that may disproportionately affect certain populations.

- **Case Studies of Vaccine Mandates in Practice**

  - Analysis of real-world examples, including school vaccine requirements, healthcare worker mandates, and travel vaccination policies.

  - Comparing outcomes of mandated versus voluntary vaccination programs in terms of coverage rates and public health impact.

  - Lessons learned from past implementations, including the challenges of enforcing mandates and balancing them with personal rights.

- **Non-Coercive Alternatives to Mandates**

  o Evaluating alternatives like educational campaigns, incentives, and voluntary vaccination programs aimed at achieving high vaccine uptake without mandates.

  o The role of persuasion, communication, and trust-building in encouraging vaccination without compulsion.

  o Studies on the effectiveness of non-coercive approaches and whether they can achieve similar outcomes to mandates in terms of vaccination rates.

This chapter offers readers an in-depth analysis of the complex ethical landscape surrounding vaccine mandates, providing insights into the motivations, challenges, and consequences of enforcing vaccination as a public health strategy.

The Role of Misinformation in the Vaccine Debate

- **Defining Misinformation and Disinformation**

  o Exploring the distinction between misinformation (false or inaccurate information spread unintentionally) and disinformation (deliberately false information spread to deceive).

- o Understanding how both types of false information impact the public's understanding of vaccines and vaccination programs.

- o The rise of misinformation in the digital age, especially through social media, and its effect on public perceptions of vaccine safety and efficacy.

- **The Spread of Vaccine Misinformation**

  - o How misinformation about vaccines spreads through traditional media, social media platforms, and word of mouth.

  - o Identifying common sources of misinformation, including celebrities, social media influencers, and websites that promote anti-vaccine rhetoric.

  - o Case studies of viral misinformation campaigns, such as the false claim that vaccines cause autism, and how they have influenced vaccine hesitancy.

- **Psychological Mechanisms Behind Vaccine Misinformation**

  - o The cognitive biases that make people more susceptible to believing and spreading vaccine misinformation, such as confirmation bias (the tendency to seek information that confirms preexisting beliefs) and availability bias (relying on easily recalled information, even if it's misleading).

- o How emotional appeals, fear, and distrust of authorities contribute to the spread of misinformation.

- o The role of social media algorithms in reinforcing misinformation, creating echo chambers that amplify misleading vaccine-related claims.

- **The Impact of Vaccine Misinformation on Public Health**

  - o Examining the real-world consequences of vaccine misinformation, including outbreaks of preventable diseases, decreased vaccination rates, and the erosion of trust in health authorities.

  - o Understanding how misinformation fuels vaccine hesitancy and refusal, and how these attitudes threaten herd immunity and community protection.

  - o Discussing the moral and ethical responsibilities of health organizations, the media, and individuals in preventing the spread of misinformation.

- **Case Studies of Misinformation in Vaccine Debates**

  - o The 1998 study by Andrew Wakefield linking the MMR vaccine to autism, which was later discredited but continued to fuel vaccine fears.

- o Misinformation surrounding the COVID-19 vaccines, including false claims about the speed of development, safety concerns, and misinformation regarding side effects.

- o The role of "anti-vax" groups and websites that perpetuate false narratives about vaccines, often using pseudoscience to bolster their claims.

- **The Role of Social Media in Amplifying Vaccine Misinformation**

  - o How platforms like Facebook, Twitter, Instagram, and YouTube have been used to spread vaccine misinformation, with algorithms amplifying false claims through engagement metrics (likes, shares, comments).

  - o The rise of anti-vaccine groups and influencers on social media and their ability to reach large audiences, particularly parents and vulnerable populations.

  - o Examining the responsibility of social media companies in curbing the spread of misinformation and the effectiveness of their efforts to fact-check, flag, or remove false vaccine-related content.

- **The Role of Traditional Media in Vaccine Misinformation**

  o How some mainstream media outlets contribute to the spread of vaccine misinformation, whether intentionally or unintentionally, through sensationalized reporting, lack of fact-checking, or providing platforms for anti-vaccine advocates.

  o Analyzing the influence of documentaries, news programs, and publications that present misleading or unbalanced views on vaccine safety.

  o The importance of responsible journalism in shaping public opinion about vaccines and maintaining trust in the scientific community.

- **The Psychological and Sociological Impact of Misinformation**

  o The psychological effects of misinformation, including fear, confusion, and distrust, which can undermine individuals' willingness to trust health authorities and follow public health recommendations.

  o How misinformation fosters social division and can polarize public opinion on vaccination, making it more difficult to achieve consensus or promote collaborative public health efforts.

- The role of echo chambers and information silos in reinforcing misinformation and making it harder for individuals to encounter reliable, fact-based information.

- **Combating Vaccine Misinformation**

    - Strategies for countering vaccine misinformation, including the role of public health campaigns, fact-checking organizations, and scientific communities in providing accurate information.

    - The importance of transparent communication from health officials, addressing concerns in a clear and empathetic manner, and correcting misinformation without alienating individuals.

    - Engaging with vaccine-hesitant individuals in a way that fosters dialogue and trust, as opposed to dismissing or antagonizing them, to encourage informed decision-making.

    - The potential of social media and digital tools to combat misinformation, including the use of influencers, celebrities, and trusted community figures to spread accurate information and debunk myths.

- **Education as a Long-Term Solution to Misinformation**

- The role of education in building scientific literacy and critical thinking skills, empowering individuals to better evaluate vaccine-related information.

- Teaching children and young adults the importance of evidence-based science and the scientific method as a means to inoculate against misinformation.

- Collaboration between healthcare providers, educators, and public health officials to create lasting educational initiatives that encourage vaccine acceptance and combat misinformation in the long run.

- **Lessons Learned from the Fight Against Vaccine Misinformation**

  - Case studies of successful interventions to reduce the spread of vaccine misinformation, such as public health campaigns during the measles outbreaks or during the COVID-19 vaccination rollout.

  - Insights into the ongoing challenges of misinformation, and what strategies can be refined or improved moving forward to protect public health.

  - The evolving landscape of vaccine communication in the digital age, and how the global community can adapt to new challenges in the fight against misinformation.

This section emphasizes the critical role misinformation plays in shaping the vaccine debate and public perception. It explores the underlying causes of vaccine misinformation, its harmful effects, and offers strategies for addressing and combating falsehoods with science, education, and transparency.

Vaccine Hesitancy and Public Trust in Health Authorities

- **Defining Vaccine Hesitancy**

  - Exploring the concept of vaccine hesitancy, a condition where individuals delay or refuse vaccination despite availability of vaccination services.

  - The spectrum of vaccine hesitancy: from complete refusal to uncertainty and delayed vaccination, and how these attitudes vary across different populations.

  - The impact of vaccine hesitancy on public health, particularly in terms of reducing herd immunity and the resurgence of preventable diseases.

- **Understanding the Causes of Vaccine Hesitancy**

  - **Mistrust in Health Authorities**: The role of historical events, past medical injustices, and perceived lack of transparency that have led to mistrust in government health agencies, such as the CDC, WHO, and FDA.

- **Perceived Risks vs. Benefits**: How individuals weigh the perceived risks of vaccination against its benefits. This includes concerns about safety, side effects, and doubts about vaccine efficacy.

- **Cultural and Socioeconomic Factors**: Examining how cultural beliefs, socioeconomic status, education levels, and access to healthcare influence vaccine attitudes. For example, marginalized communities may have lower vaccination rates due to historical mistreatment or lack of trust in modern medicine.

- **Influence of Media and Social Networks**: The role of media, both traditional and social, in shaping perceptions of vaccines. How misinformation, sensationalist media coverage, and personal stories can amplify fears and doubts.

- **Political and Ideological Factors**: How vaccine acceptance can be influenced by political beliefs, ideology, and the polarization of public health issues. Vaccine mandates, government interventions, and freedom of choice are often framed as ideological battles in the public discourse.

- **The Psychology of Vaccine Hesitancy**

  - **Cognitive Biases and Heuristics**: Understanding psychological factors that contribute to vaccine hesitancy, such as confirmation bias (the tendency to seek out information that confirms preexisting beliefs) and the availability heuristic (relying on personal experiences or highly publicized cases of adverse events to form opinions).

- **The Role of Fear and Anxiety**: How fear, whether rational or irrational, plays a central role in vaccine hesitancy. Individuals may fear adverse effects, the unknown, or being subjected to mandates, which leads to avoidance behavior.

- **Social Identity and Group Influence**: Examining how social networks, peer groups, and cultural identity influence vaccine decisions. People are often influenced by the opinions of those around them, particularly in close-knit communities or online groups where vaccine misinformation can thrive.

- **Impact of Vaccine Hesitancy on Public Health**

  - **Decreased Immunization Rates**: The direct effect of vaccine hesitancy on immunization rates, leading to pockets of unvaccinated individuals and outbreaks of vaccine-preventable diseases like measles, polio, and pertussis.

  - **Increased Vulnerability for Vulnerable Populations**: How vaccine hesitancy puts vulnerable populations, such as newborns, elderly individuals, and immunocompromised individuals, at greater risk of contracting diseases that could be prevented through vaccination.

- **The Role of Vaccine Hesitancy in Undermining Herd Immunity**: Understanding the importance of high vaccination coverage in preventing the spread of diseases and how vaccine hesitancy undermines this protective effect, leading to higher rates of infection and mortality.

- **Public Trust in Health Authorities**

  - **The Erosion of Trust in Institutions**: Exploring how decades of skepticism towards government and public health institutions have contributed to a growing divide between the public and health authorities. This erosion of trust can result from perceived inconsistencies in public health messaging, lack of transparency, or past public health failures.

  - **The Role of Health Authorities in Building Trust**: How health authorities can rebuild trust by being transparent, consistent, and responsive in their communication. This includes acknowledging mistakes, sharing data openly, and engaging in two-way communication with the public.

  - **The Importance of Transparency**: How clear, consistent, and evidence-based communication can mitigate concerns and reduce vaccine hesitancy. Transparent discussions about the safety and efficacy of vaccines, as well as the decision-making processes behind vaccination policies, can restore public confidence.

- **Addressing Historical Injustices**: The importance of addressing past historical injustices (e.g., the Tuskegee Syphilis Study, forced sterilizations, exploitation of marginalized populations) that contribute to deep-seated mistrust of healthcare systems in specific communities.

- **Strategies for Overcoming Vaccine Hesitancy**

  - **Engaging with Hesitant Populations**: How to engage individuals who are hesitant about vaccines by understanding their concerns, providing tailored information, and offering empathetic communication. Personalized conversations with healthcare providers can help clarify misconceptions and provide reassurance.

  - **Leveraging Trusted Messengers**: Using trusted community leaders, such as doctors, religious figures, local influencers, and peers, to convey accurate information and counter misinformation. Trusted individuals who share the same values as the target audience are more likely to influence vaccine decisions.

  - **Educational Campaigns and Public Health Initiatives**: Designing effective educational campaigns that focus on increasing vaccine literacy and addressing specific concerns. These campaigns should be culturally sensitive, multilingual, and targeted to reach specific communities most affected by vaccine hesitancy.

- **Incentives and Policies**: Exploring the role of policies, such as vaccine mandates, as well as incentives (e.g., financial support for vaccination, free vaccination clinics) to encourage vaccine uptake, particularly among hesitant individuals.

- **Correcting Misinformation and Disinformation**: Collaborating with media outlets, fact-checkers, and social media platforms to correct vaccine misinformation in real time. This may include debunking myths, providing evidence-based answers to common questions, and actively monitoring the spread of disinformation.

- **The Role of Public Health Campaigns in Restoring Confidence**

  - **Building Resilient Public Health Systems**: How strengthening the healthcare infrastructure, improving access to vaccinations, and offering education on vaccines can help restore confidence in health authorities.

  - **Fostering Community Engagement**: Encouraging community participation and open dialogues about vaccines can help restore trust in health systems. Building relationships with local communities and respecting their cultural values are vital for overcoming vaccine hesitancy.

- **Learning from Past Public Health Successes**: Drawing lessons from past public health campaigns, such as the polio vaccination campaign, that successfully increased public trust and achieved high vaccination rates. Understanding what worked in the past can inform future efforts to tackle vaccine hesitancy.

- **The Future of Vaccine Hesitancy and Trust**

  - **Adapting to Changing Public Sentiment**: Understanding how vaccine hesitancy may evolve over time and how health authorities can adapt their strategies to meet new challenges and concerns.

  - **Global Perspectives on Vaccine Hesitancy**: Examining vaccine hesitancy in different cultural, geographic, and political contexts, and understanding how global events (e.g., pandemics) affect vaccine attitudes across the world.

  - **Sustaining Long-Term Public Trust**: Ensuring that trust in vaccines and public health systems is maintained over the long term, through continual education, transparent practices, and by reinforcing the collective benefits of vaccination for public health.

Chapter 8: The Global Vaccine Debate: Perspectives from Different Countries

Vaccine Policies Around the World: A Comparative Overview

Vaccine policies around the world vary significantly, influenced by factors such as cultural beliefs, healthcare infrastructure, political climate, and public health priorities. This section will examine the different approaches to vaccination policies, comparing the strategies and practices adopted by various countries to address public health challenges through immunization.

- **Mandatory vs. Voluntary Vaccination**

  - **Mandatory Vaccination**: Some countries have adopted laws that require certain vaccinations for entry into school, healthcare facilities, or for employment in high-risk sectors. Countries such as **France, Italy, and Australia** have enacted strict vaccine mandates, particularly in response to disease outbreaks like measles, polio, and COVID-19. These policies often include penalties for non-compliance, such as fines or exclusion from public services.

- **Example**: In **France**, the government mandated 11 vaccines for children entering school in 2018, following a rise in vaccine-preventable diseases.

- **Australia** has a "no jab, no pay" policy, where parents who choose not to vaccinate their children can face the loss of government benefits.

  o **Voluntary Vaccination**: In contrast, countries like the **United States, Sweden, and the United Kingdom** generally adopt a voluntary approach to vaccination, where citizens are encouraged but not required to vaccinate. In these countries, health authorities focus on education and public awareness campaigns to improve vaccine uptake.

  - **Example**: In **the United States**, vaccination is largely voluntary, though some states have laws requiring vaccinations for school entry. The approach has led to varied vaccination rates, particularly in regions with strong anti-vaccine sentiments.

- **National Immunization Schedules**

  o Different countries have their own national immunization schedules based on the diseases prevalent in their regions, healthcare priorities, and the availability of vaccines.

- **United States**: The U.S. Centers for Disease Control and Prevention (CDC) provides a comprehensive immunization schedule for children, recommending vaccines for diseases such as measles, mumps, rubella (MMR), and polio. The schedule also includes vaccines for adolescents and adults, such as the HPV vaccine and annual flu shots.

- **India**: The immunization schedule in India is shaped by the prevalence of diseases like tuberculosis (TB), polio, and hepatitis B. The Indian government launched the **Universal Immunization Program** to provide vaccines for infants and young children against preventable diseases.

- **South Africa**: The South African immunization schedule includes vaccines for diseases like polio, rotavirus, and tuberculosis, with an emphasis on reaching children in rural and underserved areas through outreach programs.

- **Vaccine Access and Equity**

  o **High-Income Countries**: In many high-income countries, vaccines are widely available and provided free of charge to the population through national health systems or insurance. These countries generally have high vaccination coverage due to robust healthcare infrastructure and funding.

    ▪ **Example**: In **Canada**, vaccines are provided through provincial healthcare programs, ensuring that all citizens have access to recommended vaccinations.

  o **Low- and Middle-Income Countries**: Access to vaccines in low- and middle-income countries is often hindered by issues such as cost, distribution challenges, and limited healthcare infrastructure. However, organizations like the **Global Alliance for Vaccines and Immunization (GAVI)** and **UNICEF** have made significant strides in improving vaccine access and affordability.

    ▪ **Example**: In **Nigeria**, although vaccines are available through government and international aid programs, challenges such as logistical difficulties in remote areas, vaccine hesitancy, and political instability have impacted vaccine delivery.

- **Public Health Campaigns and Education**

  o In some countries, public health authorities actively promote vaccination through educational campaigns, mass media, and public service announcements. These efforts aim to raise awareness about the benefits of vaccination and address vaccine misconceptions.

    - **Example**: In **Mexico**, the government has carried out extensive campaigns to vaccinate against influenza, particularly targeting high-risk groups such as the elderly and those with underlying health conditions.

    - **Example**: **Sweden** is known for its strong public health education programs, which have contributed to high vaccine acceptance rates. The Swedish government utilizes a mix of traditional media, digital platforms, and outreach efforts in communities with lower vaccination rates.

- **Vaccine Distribution and Cold Chain Logistics**

  o Effective vaccine distribution is a critical component of any vaccination policy. In wealthier nations, vaccines are generally stored and transported under optimal conditions. However, in low-resource settings, maintaining the cold chain (the temperature-controlled supply chain) can be a major challenge, leading to potential wastage or compromised vaccine efficacy.

- **Example**: In **Sub-Saharan Africa**, maintaining the cold chain is a persistent issue, and the region has faced challenges in ensuring vaccines, such as those for measles and polio, are delivered and stored properly.

- **Example**: The **GAVI Alliance** has worked with countries to improve vaccine distribution by supporting cold chain infrastructure, helping to ensure vaccines reach even the most remote regions.

- **Vaccine Hesitancy and Public Resistance**

  o **Vaccine hesitancy**—the reluctance or refusal to vaccinate despite availability of vaccination services—has become a growing concern in many countries. This phenomenon is influenced by cultural, social, political, and economic factors, and it has been linked to misinformation, mistrust of health authorities, and fears about vaccine safety.

- **Example**: In **Italy**, a rise in vaccine hesitancy led to the implementation of a stricter vaccine mandate for school-aged children. Despite this, some communities remain resistant, driven by misinformation about vaccine safety and fears about government overreach.

- **Example**: In **Japan**, the government faced vaccine hesitancy during the 1990s following allegations of side effects linked to the DPT vaccine. This hesitancy contributed to a decline in vaccination rates and a resurgence of preventable diseases such as rubella and whooping cough.

- **Cultural and Religious Factors in Vaccination Policies**

  o Cultural attitudes and religious beliefs can strongly influence vaccine acceptance in different countries. In some regions, vaccination policies must navigate sensitive cultural or religious concerns to ensure broader acceptance.

    - **Example**: In **Nigeria**, certain religious groups have been resistant to polio vaccination, citing suspicions about the vaccine's safety or its alleged connection to sterilization efforts. Public health campaigns tailored to specific cultural and religious contexts have been critical in overcoming these barriers.

- **Example**: In **Saudi Arabia**, religious leaders have played a significant role in promoting vaccination, particularly among pilgrims to the Hajj, where vaccination against diseases like meningitis is required.

- **Global Cooperation and Vaccine Diplomacy**

  - **Vaccine diplomacy** refers to the use of vaccine distribution as a tool of international relations, where countries provide vaccines to others as part of foreign policy strategies. This has become especially prominent during the COVID-19 pandemic, with countries like **China** and **Russia** offering their vaccines to developing countries.

    - **Example: India** has emerged as a key player in global vaccine distribution, with the Serum Institute of India producing and distributing vaccines to many low- and middle-income countries through programs like **COVAX**.

- **Example**: **China's Sinovac vaccine** was widely distributed in countries across Latin America, Africa, and Asia, often as part of broader diplomatic efforts to strengthen ties with these regions.

- **Vaccine Innovation and Policy Adjustments**
  - As new vaccines are developed, national vaccine policies must adapt to incorporate emerging technologies and strategies for immunization.
    - **Example**: The rapid development and approval of mRNA vaccines for COVID-19 highlighted the ability of some countries to quickly adjust their vaccine policies in response to new health threats. **Israel** became a global leader in mRNA vaccine administration, with a quick rollout of the Pfizer-BioNTech vaccine and extensive data collection for future public health strategies.

In conclusion, vaccine policies worldwide reflect the diverse needs and challenges of different countries. While high-income countries often lead in vaccine coverage and innovation, low-income countries continue to face significant barriers to achieving universal vaccine access. Global cooperation, public health education, and targeted vaccine strategies are crucial to overcoming these challenges and ensuring that vaccines reach all populations, regardless of location or socioeconomic status.

How Different Nations Handle Vaccine Hesitancy

Vaccine hesitancy—the reluctance or refusal to vaccinate despite availability of vaccination services—poses a significant challenge to public health worldwide. Addressing vaccine hesitancy requires understanding the specific social, cultural, political, and informational contexts of each country. Different nations have developed various strategies to combat hesitancy, from public education campaigns to policy interventions and community engagement.

1. United States: Public Education and Engagement

In the United States, vaccine hesitancy has been a concern for several years, particularly in relation to vaccines for children, like the MMR (measles, mumps, rubella) vaccine. To address hesitancy:

- **Public Health Campaigns**: The U.S. Centers for Disease Control and Prevention (CDC) and the American Academy of Pediatrics (AAP) run extensive public education campaigns to combat misinformation and provide clear, factual information about vaccine safety.

- **Health Communication**: There has been a focus on improving communication strategies to engage communities and tailor messages that address specific concerns. Healthcare professionals play a key role in educating parents and patients, often using one-on-one consultations to counteract fears.

- **Legislation**: Some states have enacted laws requiring vaccinations for school enrollment, which has led to some improvements in vaccination rates. However, vaccine exemptions (for medical, religious, and philosophical reasons) vary across states, with some having stricter policies to limit non-vaccination.

2. United Kingdom: Building Trust Through Healthcare Providers

In the UK, vaccine hesitancy has been a concern for vaccines such as the MMR and, more recently, COVID-19 vaccines. Key approaches include:

- **Engagement with Healthcare Professionals**: The National Health Service (NHS) relies heavily on healthcare providers to encourage vaccination. Trusted figures like family doctors and pediatricians are critical in dispelling myths and answering questions about vaccines.

- **Targeted Outreach**: Specific communities, such as those with high levels of vaccine hesitancy (e.g., Black, Asian, and Minority Ethnic [BAME] communities), have been targeted with tailored messages and outreach programs.

- **Public Campaigns**: During the COVID-19 pandemic, the UK government launched national campaigns, including advertising on television, social media, and in public spaces, to encourage vaccination. The messaging emphasized the safety and importance of vaccination, particularly to protect vulnerable groups.

3. Australia: Policy Mandates and Public Awareness

Australia has been proactive in tackling vaccine hesitancy, particularly with the **"No Jab, No Pay"** policy, which links vaccination to government benefits. This approach includes:

- **No Jab, No Pay**: This policy cuts government financial support for parents who refuse to vaccinate their children. This strategy has proven effective in increasing vaccination rates, particularly for childhood immunizations.

- **Education and Awareness**: The Australian government has launched several public health campaigns to educate people on the safety and benefits of vaccines. These campaigns are designed to target individuals and communities with the lowest vaccination rates, including regional and remote populations.

- **Targeted Programs for Vulnerable Groups**: Indigenous populations and rural communities have been the focus of outreach efforts, ensuring that vaccines are accessible and culturally sensitive information is provided.

4. France: Legal Mandates and Public Dialogue

In France, vaccine hesitancy is a significant issue, with skepticism about vaccine safety and government mandates being widespread. To address this:

- **Mandatory Vaccines for Children**: In 2018, France expanded its vaccine mandate, requiring children to receive 11 vaccines before enrolling in school. This was part of a broader effort to combat vaccine hesitancy and protect public health from preventable diseases like measles.

- **Building Public Dialogue**: French authorities have worked to create transparent, open conversations about the safety of vaccines. Public health bodies collaborate with independent experts to provide evidence-based information and counter vaccine misinformation.

- **Increased Funding for Information Campaigns**: France has invested in public health campaigns, utilizing various media platforms to reassure the public about the benefits of vaccines, particularly in light of the 2018 measles outbreak.

5. Sweden: Respecting Autonomy and Trust in Public Health Systems

Sweden's approach to vaccine hesitancy has been relatively successful, largely due to the strong trust that the population places in the country's public health system.

- **Voluntary Vaccination Policy**: Sweden does not mandate vaccinations, but the high level of public trust in the healthcare system means that vaccine hesitancy is lower compared to many other countries.

- **Health System Trust**: Efforts focus on ensuring that the population continues to trust health authorities. The Swedish government and public health officials work hard to provide clear, science-backed information, particularly during times of vaccine-related controversies.

- **Engaging Communities**: Sweden has also implemented targeted communication efforts to address concerns in communities with higher rates of vaccine hesitancy, such as immigrant populations.

6. Italy: Vaccine Mandates and Public Health Campaigns

Italy, like other European countries, has faced challenges in vaccine acceptance, particularly after concerns over the safety of vaccines were amplified in the media.

- **Strict Vaccine Mandates**: In response to declining vaccination rates and rising cases of measles, Italy implemented a law in 2017 that made 10 vaccines mandatory for children attending school. This policy helped to increase vaccination rates and curb outbreaks.

- **Public Health Campaigns**: The Italian Ministry of Health launched public campaigns focusing on the importance of vaccination. These campaigns highlighted the risks of preventable diseases and the benefits of immunization, using a mix of traditional media, social media, and community outreach.

- **Rebuilding Public Trust**: Efforts have been made to rebuild public trust in vaccines through increased transparency, collaboration with pediatricians and family doctors, and addressing misinformation.

7. Nigeria: Combating Misinformation and Cultural Resistance

In Nigeria, vaccine hesitancy has been particularly challenging due to cultural beliefs, religious opposition, and misinformation.

- **Community Engagement**: The government and international organizations like **WHO** and **UNICEF** have focused on engaging local communities to improve understanding and acceptance of vaccines, particularly in rural and nomadic populations. These efforts involve working with community leaders and religious figures to promote vaccines as a health measure.

- **Combating Misinformation**: A significant effort has been made to counter misinformation about vaccines, particularly concerning the polio vaccine, which faced resistance due to false rumors. Public health messages have been tailored to address these specific concerns and present clear, accurate information.

- **Global Partnerships**: Nigeria has worked with global health organizations to ensure vaccines are accessible, even in remote regions, and to facilitate education about vaccine safety.

8. India: Grassroots Outreach and Addressing Cultural Barriers

India faces significant challenges related to vaccine hesitancy, especially in rural areas and among marginalized populations.

- **Grassroots Mobilization**: The government has used grassroots programs to educate communities about the benefits of vaccination. Local health workers, including community health volunteers, play a key role in delivering information and addressing concerns in culturally sensitive ways.

- **Targeted Communication**: To overcome hesitancy, India has tailored messaging for different demographic groups, focusing on the safety and efficacy of vaccines while addressing common fears. The government works with trusted community figures to help change attitudes.

- **Expanding Access**: India's immunization programs have expanded to rural and underserved populations, using mobile vaccination units and outreach campaigns to ensure that vaccines reach those who are most hesitant or difficult to reach.

9. Japan: Overcoming Historical Distrust in Vaccines

Japan's experience with vaccine hesitancy is shaped by historical events, such as the controversy over side effects linked to the DPT (diphtheria, pertussis, tetanus) vaccine in the 1970s.

- **Building Trust**: The Japanese government has worked to rebuild trust in vaccines by providing thorough, scientifically backed explanations of vaccine safety. Public health officials continue to engage with the public to explain the benefits of immunization.

- **Education and Transparency**: Japan focuses on providing clear, transparent information about vaccine side effects and benefits. There is also a strong emphasis on educating the population to prevent the spread of misinformation.

10. Brazil: Combating Misinformation and Strengthening Vaccination Programs

Brazil has experienced high levels of vaccine acceptance, but recent rises in vaccine hesitancy, particularly for the measles vaccine, have prompted the government to take action.

- **National Vaccination Campaigns**: Brazil has launched national vaccination campaigns to address declining vaccination rates, especially in urban areas where misinformation about vaccines is more prevalent.

- **Social Media Engagement**: The Brazilian government has used social media to engage the public, providing accurate information about vaccines and combating myths.

- **Mobile Clinics and Outreach**: Mobile vaccination units are deployed in areas with low vaccination coverage, helping to overcome logistical barriers and ensure that people receive vaccines.

Conclusion: A Global Challenge, Diverse Solutions

Handling vaccine hesitancy requires a multifaceted approach, involving government policy, public health communication, community engagement, and addressing misinformation. Countries like the United States, the UK, and France have emphasized education and public campaigns, while others, like Australia and Italy, have utilized mandates to encourage vaccination. Understanding the unique challenges and cultural contexts of each nation is crucial for successfully addressing vaccine hesitancy and ensuring that immunization efforts are both effective and widely accepted.

The Role of Global Organizations: WHO, GAVI, and UNICEF in Vaccine Distribution

Global health organizations play an essential role in addressing vaccine hesitancy, ensuring equitable access to vaccines, and facilitating large-scale vaccination efforts worldwide. Among the most prominent organizations in vaccine distribution are the **World Health Organization (WHO)**, the **Global Alliance for Vaccines and Immunization (GAVI)**, and **UNICEF**. Each of these entities has unique responsibilities and approaches, but all are united in their mission to promote health through immunization and to ensure that vaccines reach the most vulnerable populations around the world.

1. World Health Organization (WHO)

The **World Health Organization (WHO)** is the leading international body in global health governance. It coordinates efforts between governments, health agencies, and other stakeholders to address major health issues, including vaccine-preventable diseases.

- **Global Health Standards and Guidelines**: WHO sets the standards for vaccine quality, safety, and efficacy through rigorous scientific review. It provides guidelines for vaccine production, distribution, and administration, ensuring that vaccines are of high quality and safe for public use.

- **Immunization Programs**: WHO leads global vaccination initiatives, such as the **Expanded Programme on Immunization (EPI)**, which aims to ensure that all children, regardless of where they live, receive critical vaccines. The WHO also works with national governments to strengthen immunization systems and tackle vaccine hesitancy.

- **Polio Eradication**: The **Global Polio Eradication Initiative (GPEI)**, spearheaded by WHO, has been a key effort in reducing polio worldwide. WHO has played a critical role in coordinating vaccination campaigns, monitoring disease outbreaks, and working with local health authorities to ensure effective vaccination strategies.

- **Emergency Response**: WHO is at the forefront of emergency vaccination campaigns, such as those for outbreaks of **Ebola, cholera,** and **COVID-19**. It coordinates rapid response efforts, ensures vaccines are distributed where they are most needed, and provides technical support to affected countries.

- **Vaccine Access in Low-Resource Settings**: WHO works with governments and partners to improve vaccination coverage in low-income and remote areas. It also addresses logistical challenges in vaccine distribution, such as cold-chain infrastructure and access to transportation.

2. Global Alliance for Vaccines and Immunization (GAVI)

GAVI, founded in 2000, is a public-private partnership aimed at increasing access to vaccines in developing countries. GAVI plays a crucial role in ensuring that vaccines are affordable and accessible to people who need them the most.

- **Equitable Vaccine Access**: One of GAVI's main goals is to make vaccines more affordable and accessible to low-income countries, where the burden of vaccine-preventable diseases is often highest. GAVI works with manufacturers to secure discounted vaccine prices and to negotiate global procurement deals.

- **Financing and Subsidies**: GAVI mobilizes financial resources from governments, philanthropic foundations, and private sector partners to fund immunization programs. Through these funds, GAVI provides subsidies to countries so that vaccines are free or heavily discounted for the most vulnerable populations, including children and pregnant women.

- **Vaccine Supply and Procurement**: GAVI coordinates the global procurement and distribution of vaccines, ensuring that countries receive the vaccines they need in a timely manner. GAVI also works on improving vaccine supply chains, ensuring vaccines are delivered effectively and efficiently to remote regions.

- **Technical Assistance and Capacity Building**: GAVI provides technical assistance to countries, helping them to strengthen their immunization systems and infrastructure. This includes training healthcare workers, improving data collection, and establishing efficient delivery systems to ensure vaccines reach every community.

- **Support for New and Innovative Vaccines**: GAVI is also instrumental in supporting the development and introduction of new vaccines, such as those for **HPV (human papillomavirus)** and **pneumococcal disease**. The organization works to ensure these vaccines are made available to the populations most in need.

- **Strengthening Routine Immunization**: GAVI supports governments in strengthening their routine immunization programs. This includes funding national vaccination campaigns, improving vaccine supply systems, and building trust in vaccination services.

3. UNICEF

UNICEF, the United Nations Children's Fund, is another critical organization involved in global vaccine distribution. UNICEF has a particular focus on children's health and plays an essential role in immunization efforts worldwide.

- **Vaccine Distribution**: UNICEF is one of the largest procurers and distributors of vaccines globally, ensuring that millions of children in low- and middle-income countries receive routine vaccinations. UNICEF works closely with governments, the WHO, and GAVI to ensure vaccines reach every child, regardless of geographic location or socio-economic status.

- **Cold Chain and Logistics**: UNICEF is responsible for setting up and maintaining the global cold-chain system, which ensures that vaccines are stored and transported at the proper temperature to maintain their efficacy. This infrastructure is especially critical in tropical and remote areas, where access to reliable electricity and refrigeration can be challenging.

- **Emergency Vaccine Delivery**: In situations of humanitarian crises, such as in conflict zones or during natural disasters, UNICEF plays a vital role in delivering vaccines and organizing immunization campaigns. This includes vaccinating against diseases like measles and polio, which can spread rapidly in crowded refugee camps or post-disaster areas.

- **Education and Advocacy**: UNICEF engages in public awareness campaigns to educate families about the importance of vaccines. It collaborates with governments to promote vaccine acceptance and counter misinformation, which is crucial in combating vaccine hesitancy.

- **Maternal and Child Health Programs**: In addition to childhood immunization, UNICEF works to improve maternal health by promoting the vaccination of women, particularly during pregnancy, to protect both mothers and their newborns from preventable diseases.

- **Strengthening Health Systems**: UNICEF helps countries build their healthcare infrastructure, including vaccination delivery systems, healthcare worker training, and improving vaccine monitoring. This is essential for increasing immunization coverage and achieving long-term health goals.

Collaboration Between WHO, GAVI, and UNICEF

The combined efforts of WHO, GAVI, and UNICEF are essential in tackling global vaccine inequities. These organizations collaborate on various initiatives and share resources to maximize their impact.

- **COVAX Initiative**: A prime example of their collaboration is the **COVAX initiative**, led by WHO, GAVI, and other global partners, which was created to ensure equitable access to COVID-19 vaccines worldwide. COVAX works to procure and distribute vaccines to low- and middle-income countries, with the goal of making vaccines accessible to all countries, regardless of their wealth.

- **Global Immunization Strategies**: WHO, GAVI, and UNICEF align their strategies and priorities to support global immunization goals, such as the **Global Vaccine Safety Initiative**, the **Measles and Rubella Elimination Strategy**, and the **Global Polio Eradication Initiative**. These initiatives aim to eliminate vaccine-preventable diseases and increase global immunization coverage.

- **Funding and Advocacy**: Through their partnerships, these organizations mobilize financial support for immunization programs, advocate for greater investments in vaccines, and work with governments to prioritize vaccines in national health plans.

Challenges Faced by Global Organizations in Vaccine Distribution

Despite their critical roles, global organizations face several challenges in vaccine distribution:

- **Supply Chain and Infrastructure Issues**: Cold chain logistics and transportation infrastructure remain significant challenges, especially in conflict zones, remote rural areas, and during times of crisis.

- **Vaccine Hesitancy**: Misinformation, cultural barriers, and distrust in vaccines persist in many countries, making it difficult to achieve widespread vaccine coverage.

- **Funding and Resource Allocation**: Securing sufficient funding to support vaccine procurement, distribution, and public health initiatives is an ongoing challenge, particularly during economic downturns or competing health priorities.

- **Political and Social Barriers**: Political instability, conflict, and social unrest can disrupt vaccination campaigns and prevent access to vulnerable populations.

Conclusion

WHO, GAVI, and UNICEF play indispensable roles in global vaccine distribution, working together to ensure that vaccines are accessible, safe, and effective for everyone, particularly in low- and middle-income countries. Their coordinated efforts have been key to advancing immunization programs worldwide, contributing to the reduction of vaccine-preventable diseases, and helping to save millions of lives. However, challenges remain, and continued global cooperation is essential to achieving the ultimate goal of universal vaccine access and protection against preventable diseases.

Addressing Vaccine Inequity and Access in Developing Countries

Vaccine inequity remains one of the most pressing challenges in global health, with large disparities in access to vaccines between high-income and low- and middle-income countries. While vaccines have proven to be one of the most effective tools in preventing infectious diseases, millions of people in developing countries still lack access to life-saving vaccines. Addressing vaccine inequity is crucial not only for improving individual health but also for protecting global public health and ensuring that no one is left behind in the fight against vaccine-preventable diseases.

1. The Global Vaccine Access Problem

In many developing countries, vaccine access is hindered by a variety of factors, including **financial constraints**, **limited infrastructure**, **geographic isolation**, **political instability**, and **health system weaknesses**. These challenges prevent vaccines from reaching the populations that need them most. The COVID-19 pandemic further highlighted these disparities, as wealthy nations secured vaccine supplies in advance, leaving low-income countries to struggle with insufficient access.

- **Cost of Vaccines**: Many vaccines are expensive, and developing countries often cannot afford to purchase them in the quantities required to meet the needs of their populations. While some vaccines are subsidized or provided through initiatives like GAVI, many countries still face difficulties with procurement, particularly for newer or specialized vaccines.

- **Weak Healthcare Infrastructure**: In low-resource settings, healthcare infrastructure is often inadequate to support effective vaccine distribution. This includes a lack of reliable transportation networks, insufficient cold-chain systems to store and transport vaccines, and shortages of trained healthcare workers to administer vaccines.

- **Geographic Barriers**: Remote and rural communities in developing countries often face significant barriers to accessing health services, including vaccines. Poor road networks, long distances, and lack of local health facilities make it difficult for people to receive immunizations.

- **Political and Social Barriers**: In regions of conflict, political instability, or social unrest, vaccine distribution efforts can be severely disrupted. Additionally, vaccine hesitancy driven by misinformation or cultural resistance can further hinder immunization efforts in certain communities.

2. Global Initiatives to Address Vaccine Inequity

Several international organizations and initiatives are working to address vaccine inequity and improve access to vaccines in developing countries. These efforts focus on increasing vaccine affordability, improving distribution networks, and strengthening health systems.

COVAX Initiative

The **COVAX initiative**, a collaboration between the **World Health Organization (WHO)**, **GAVI**, **UNICEF**, and other global partners, was created to ensure equitable access to vaccines, particularly during the COVID-19 pandemic. COVAX's mission is to ensure that vaccines are available to all countries, regardless of their income level. COVAX works by pooling resources from wealthy nations, donors, and manufacturers to secure vaccines and distribute them to low- and middle-income countries.

- **Vaccine Procurement**: Through COVAX, developing countries receive vaccines at no or low cost, enabling them to vaccinate their populations without the burden of full payment.

- **Equitable Distribution**: The COVAX facility aims to distribute vaccines based on need rather than purchasing power, with priority given to frontline healthcare workers, the elderly, and high-risk populations in developing countries.

- **Supply Chain Support**: COVAX also provides technical support to strengthen cold-chain logistics and distribution networks, ensuring that vaccines reach remote areas in good condition.

GAVI (Global Alliance for Vaccines and Immunization)

GAVI plays a key role in improving vaccine access in developing countries by working with governments, vaccine manufacturers, and donors to ensure affordable and equitable access to vaccines.

- **Financial Support**: GAVI provides funding to countries to help them procure vaccines and strengthen their vaccination programs. This support enables countries to introduce new vaccines and expand immunization coverage.

- **Vaccine Price Negotiation**: GAVI negotiates with vaccine manufacturers to secure discounted prices for vaccines, making them more affordable for low-income countries. This helps to reduce the financial burden on national health budgets.

- **Health System Strengthening**: In addition to vaccine distribution, GAVI works to strengthen healthcare infrastructure in developing countries. This includes improving cold-chain storage systems, training healthcare workers, and developing better data collection and surveillance systems to track vaccination coverage and prevent outbreaks.

- **Country Tailored Approaches**: GAVI works closely with countries to develop tailored vaccination strategies that address specific health challenges and local barriers to access, including logistical constraints, political instability, and cultural factors.

UNICEF's Role

UNICEF plays a critical role in ensuring vaccines reach children in the most vulnerable and underserved regions of the world.

- **Vaccine Procurement and Distribution**: UNICEF is one of the largest buyers and distributors of vaccines globally. It works with countries, manufacturers, and other partners to ensure that vaccines are delivered where they are most needed, especially in conflict zones and rural areas.

- **Cold Chain and Logistics**: UNICEF has a robust cold-chain logistics system that ensures vaccines are stored and transported under the proper conditions. In many developing countries, UNICEF's cold-chain system is essential for maintaining the potency of vaccines, particularly those that require refrigeration.

- **Emergency Vaccine Response**: UNICEF is often at the forefront of emergency vaccination efforts during outbreaks of diseases such as polio, measles, and cholera. In crisis situations, UNICEF works to ensure vaccines are delivered quickly to prevent further spread.

- **Advocacy and Education**: UNICEF advocates for increased funding for immunization and raises awareness about the importance of vaccines in preventing diseases. It also works to combat vaccine hesitancy through education campaigns, especially in countries where distrust of vaccines is a barrier to access.

3. Innovative Approaches to Overcome Barriers

In addition to the efforts of global organizations, there are several innovative approaches to address the barriers to vaccine access in developing countries.

- **Local Vaccine Manufacturing**: Encouraging and supporting local vaccine production in developing countries can help reduce costs and improve access. Some countries, such as India, have developed strong vaccine manufacturing capabilities that allow them to produce vaccines at a fraction of the cost of purchasing them from foreign suppliers. Initiatives like the **Africa CDC** are working to increase vaccine production capacity across Africa to ensure self-sufficiency and improve local access.

- **Mobile Vaccination Clinics**: To address geographic barriers, mobile vaccination clinics can be deployed to reach remote and underserved populations. These clinics can provide vaccines in hard-to-reach areas where health facilities may be scarce.

- **Community Health Workers**: Empowering local community health workers to deliver vaccines can be an effective way to reach populations in rural and marginalized areas. Training community health workers to provide immunizations helps build trust and ensures that vaccines are delivered in a culturally appropriate manner.

- **Public-Private Partnerships**: Collaborations between governments, non-governmental organizations, and private companies can help overcome financial and logistical barriers to vaccine access. These partnerships often focus on reducing vaccine costs, improving distribution, and increasing local production capacity.

- **Incentivizing Vaccine Uptake**: Some countries have introduced innovative strategies to incentivize vaccine uptake, such as cash transfers, health insurance coverage, and other incentives for families who vaccinate their children. These programs can help improve vaccine coverage and encourage hesitant populations to get vaccinated.

4. Addressing Vaccine Hesitancy in Developing Countries

Vaccine hesitancy is a significant barrier to vaccine access in many developing countries. Misinformation, cultural beliefs, and mistrust in government or healthcare systems can prevent people from seeking vaccines for themselves or their children.

- **Community Engagement**: Community engagement and education are essential for addressing vaccine hesitancy. Engaging trusted local leaders, religious figures, and community influencers can help combat misinformation and promote the benefits of vaccination.

- **Cultural Sensitivity**: Vaccine campaigns must be culturally sensitive and take into account the beliefs and concerns of local populations. This includes addressing specific fears and misconceptions about vaccines and tailoring communication strategies to local contexts.

- **Media and Social Media**: Leveraging traditional media, as well as social media platforms, to spread accurate information about vaccines is critical in combating vaccine hesitancy. Global organizations can collaborate with local media outlets to promote positive messages about immunization and counter false claims.

5. Conclusion

Vaccine inequity remains a major global health challenge, but through international collaboration, innovative solutions, and sustained investment in health infrastructure, progress is being made. The efforts of organizations like WHO, GAVI, UNICEF, and COVAX are critical in ensuring that vaccines reach the most vulnerable populations. However, addressing the barriers to vaccine access requires continued global cooperation, investment in local health systems, and targeted interventions to address both logistical and social barriers. Only by overcoming these challenges can we ensure that vaccines are accessible to all and that we make progress toward global health equity.

Chapter 9: The Future of Vaccination

Advancements in Vaccine Technology: mRNA, DNA, and Beyond

Vaccines have been a cornerstone of public health for decades, saving millions of lives and preventing countless diseases. However, the science behind vaccines continues to evolve, with groundbreaking advancements in technology that promise to revolutionize how vaccines are developed, administered, and distributed. Among the most significant of these advancements are **mRNA** and **DNA vaccines**, which have shown tremendous potential, particularly during the COVID-19 pandemic. Beyond these, emerging technologies like **nanoparticle vaccines**, **microneedle patches**, and **universal vaccines** are shaping the future of immunization. This section delves into these innovations, their implications for global health, and what the future holds for vaccine technology.

1. mRNA Vaccines: A Breakthrough in Vaccine Development

How mRNA Vaccines Work

The development of **mRNA vaccines** marked a transformative shift in how we approach vaccine design. Unlike traditional vaccines, which use weakened or inactivated forms of viruses to stimulate an immune response, mRNA vaccines use genetic material—messenger RNA (mRNA)—to instruct cells to produce proteins that mimic parts of a pathogen, triggering the immune system to respond.

- **Mechanism of Action**: When injected into the body, the mRNA in the vaccine instructs cells to produce a protein that is typically found on the surface of the pathogen (e.g., the spike protein of the **SARS-CoV-2** virus). The immune system recognizes this protein as foreign and mounts an immune response. This primes the immune system to recognize and fight the actual virus if the body is exposed in the future.

Advantages of mRNA Technology

- **Speed and Flexibility**: One of the key advantages of mRNA vaccines is their rapid development. Traditional vaccine development can take years, but mRNA vaccines can be designed and manufactured in a matter of months, which is crucial during pandemics. The mRNA platform is versatile and can be quickly adapted to new pathogens, offering a much faster response to emerging infectious diseases.

- **No Live Pathogens**: mRNA vaccines do not use live pathogens, which reduces the risk of causing disease in recipients. They also do not require any adjuvants (substances used to enhance the immune response), making them a simpler and safer option.

- **Potential for Broader Use**: mRNA technology is not limited to COVID-19. Research is underway to develop mRNA vaccines for a range of infectious diseases, including **HIV**, **Zika virus**, **malaria**, and **influenza**. This technology has the potential to create vaccines for diseases that have long been difficult to target with traditional methods.

Challenges and Future Prospects

- **Storage and Stability**: One of the main challenges of mRNA vaccines is their requirement for cold storage. Most mRNA vaccines need to be kept at very low temperatures, which can pose logistical challenges in low-resource settings. However, advancements in formulation and delivery methods are working to address this issue.

- **Long-term Efficacy and Safety**: While mRNA vaccines have shown impressive results in the short term, ongoing research is focused on determining their long-term safety and effectiveness. Understanding how these vaccines perform over time will be crucial for their widespread use.

2. DNA Vaccines: A Promising Alternative

How DNA Vaccines Work

DNA vaccines represent another innovative technology, utilizing **plasmid DNA** (circular DNA molecules) to introduce a piece of the pathogen's genetic material into the body. This DNA instructs the cells to produce an antigen (a protein or part of a pathogen) that triggers an immune response. DNA vaccines essentially teach the immune system to recognize and attack pathogens by encoding the relevant part of the pathogen's genome.

- **Mechanism of Action**: When administered, the DNA vaccine is taken up by cells in the body, which then use the instructions to produce the pathogen-specific protein. This protein is displayed on the surface of the cells, prompting the immune system to recognize and fight it.

Advantages of DNA Vaccines

- **Stability and Storage**: DNA vaccines are more stable than traditional vaccines and do not require refrigeration, which makes them easier to transport and store, particularly in resource-limited regions.

- **Cost-Effectiveness**: DNA vaccines can be produced at a relatively low cost compared to other vaccine technologies, making them a potentially affordable option for mass immunization campaigns, particularly in low-income countries.

- **Broad Application**: DNA vaccines can be used for a wide range of diseases, including **HIV**, **Zika virus**, and **malaria**. The technology also shows promise in cancer immunotherapy, where vaccines could be developed to target specific tumor cells.

Challenges and Future Prospects

- **Efficient Delivery**: One of the biggest challenges with DNA vaccines is ensuring the DNA reaches the right cells and is successfully incorporated into the body's cells. Current delivery methods, such as **gene gun** devices and **electroporation** (electrical pulses to facilitate DNA uptake), are being explored, but they still require refinement for broader use.

- **Immune Response**: While DNA vaccines can produce strong immune responses, enhancing their efficacy through optimized delivery mechanisms and adjuvants remains a key focus for future research.

3. Nanoparticle Vaccines: Enhancing Delivery and Efficacy

Nanotechnology has paved the way for the development of **nanoparticle vaccines**, which use tiny nanoparticles (often made of lipids, proteins, or polymers) to deliver antigens to the immune system more effectively.

How Nanoparticle Vaccines Work

- **Enhanced Immune Response**: Nanoparticles can be engineered to mimic the structure of viruses, improving the way the immune system recognizes and responds to antigens. These particles can also be designed to enhance the stability of vaccines and improve how they are delivered into cells.

- **Targeted Delivery**: Nanoparticles can be used to target specific cells or tissues in the body, providing a more controlled immune response and increasing the effectiveness of the vaccine. This ability to direct the immune system's focus could be particularly useful for challenging diseases.

Advantages of Nanoparticle Vaccines

- **Improved Stability and Storage**: Like DNA vaccines, nanoparticle vaccines can be more stable than traditional vaccines, and their delivery systems may offer more options for oral or nasal administration, reducing the need for injections.

- **Higher Efficacy**: Nanoparticles can enhance the presentation of antigens, increasing the likelihood of a strong immune response, which could result in more effective vaccines with longer-lasting protection.

4. Microneedle Vaccines: Pain-Free and Convenient

Another innovative technology in vaccine development is the **microneedle patch**, which aims to make vaccination more accessible and less painful. These patches contain tiny needles that are small enough to be almost painless when applied to the skin.

How Microneedle Vaccines Work

- **Skin-Targeted Delivery**: The microneedles create tiny channels in the skin through which the vaccine is delivered. The patches can be applied by individuals themselves, making them an ideal solution for mass immunization campaigns.

Advantages of Microneedle Vaccines

- **Ease of Use**: Microneedle patches can be self-administered, reducing the need for trained healthcare professionals to administer vaccines. This can simplify the logistics of mass vaccination programs, especially in remote areas.

- **Reduced Pain and Discomfort**: Microneedles are designed to be less painful than traditional needles, which could increase vaccine acceptance, especially among children or people with a fear of needles.

- **No Refrigeration**: Some microneedle patches do not require refrigeration, making them ideal for use in areas with limited cold-chain infrastructure.

5. Universal Vaccines: The Holy Grail of Immunization

The future of vaccination also lies in the development of **universal vaccines**, which would provide long-term protection against a wide range of pathogens, including rapidly mutating viruses like the flu and coronavirus.

Universal Influenza Vaccine

Currently, flu vaccines need to be updated annually due to the constant mutation of the influenza virus. Scientists are working on a **universal flu vaccine** that would provide protection against a broad range of flu strains and could last for several years.

Universal Coronavirus Vaccine

The development of a **universal coronavirus vaccine** that provides protection against all variants of coronaviruses, including **SARS-CoV-2**, **SARS-CoV-1**, and others, is a major goal in the field of vaccine research. Such a vaccine could prevent future pandemics and reduce the need for emergency vaccine development.

6. Conclusion: The Future is Bright

The advancements in vaccine technology, including mRNA, DNA, nanoparticles, and microneedles, are opening new frontiers in the battle against infectious diseases. These innovations promise to make vaccines more effective, accessible, and affordable, improving global health and preparing us for future health challenges. With continued research and development, vaccines will remain at the heart of public health efforts, offering hope for the prevention and eradication of diseases across the globe.

Personalized Vaccines: The Next Frontier in Immunization

The field of immunization is undergoing a revolution, with emerging technologies that allow for more tailored, effective, and precise vaccination strategies. One of the most exciting frontiers in vaccine development is the rise of **personalized vaccines**. These vaccines, designed to address an individual's unique genetic, environmental, and health profile, hold the potential to enhance the effectiveness of immunization and provide a new level of precision in preventing and treating diseases.

What Are Personalized Vaccines?

Personalized vaccines, also known as **precision vaccines**, are vaccines that are specifically designed to suit the unique characteristics of an individual's immune system. Rather than using a one-size-fits-all approach, personalized vaccines take into account an individual's genetics, medical history, lifestyle factors, and even their response to previous vaccines or infections. By targeting an individual's specific needs, these vaccines aim to optimize protection and provide a more powerful immune response.

Personalized vaccines can be developed for various medical conditions, including infectious diseases, cancer, and even autoimmune disorders. The most advanced examples are those being researched for **cancer immunotherapy** and **infectious diseases** like influenza, COVID-19, and HIV.

Key Concepts Behind Personalized Vaccines

1. Genetic Profiling and Immunogenomics

Personalized vaccines rely heavily on **genetic profiling** and **immunogenomics**, a branch of genomics focused on understanding how genes affect immune responses. Through genetic testing, scientists can identify specific genetic markers that influence how an individual's immune system will respond to pathogens or vaccine candidates. By understanding these markers, vaccines can be tailored to enhance the immune system's response, ensuring better protection against the disease.

- **Cancer Vaccines**: For example, in cancer immunotherapy, scientists study the unique mutations found in a person's cancer cells. These mutations can be used to design a personalized vaccine that targets and stimulates the immune system to attack cancer cells specifically. This approach holds promise for treating cancers that have proven difficult to treat with traditional methods, such as melanoma and non-small-cell lung cancer.

- **Infectious Disease Vaccines**: For infectious diseases like **COVID-19**, **HIV**, and **influenza**, personalized vaccines could be tailored to an individual's genetic predisposition and previous exposure. For instance, certain genetic factors may influence how a person's immune system responds to the spike protein in SARS-CoV-2, making some individuals more likely to develop severe symptoms. A personalized vaccine would aim to boost the immune response in these individuals to protect against the virus.

2. Immune System Response Mapping

The immune system varies from person to person, and factors such as **age**, **health conditions**, **hormonal differences**, and **previous infections** all influence how the body responds to pathogens. Personalized vaccines aim to map these differences and design immunization strategies that are most likely to result in a strong and effective immune response.

- **T-cell and B-cell Targeting**: Personalized vaccines could focus on stimulating specific T-

cells and **B-cells**, which are essential for adaptive immunity. By identifying the most effective T-cell and B-cell responses for an individual, the vaccine can be customized to maximize the body's natural defenses.

- **Adjuvant Optimization**: Personalized vaccines may also involve selecting the most effective **adjuvants**—substances that enhance the immune response. By understanding which adjuvants work best for each individual based on their immune profile, researchers can fine-tune vaccine formulations for more potent protection.

3. Tailoring Vaccine Platforms

Personalized vaccines might be based on various vaccine platforms, including **mRNA, DNA, protein subunit**, and **viral vector vaccines**. Each platform has its strengths and can be customized to suit an individual's immune system:

- **mRNA vaccines** can be adapted relatively easily for personalized medicine. For example, in the case of cancer, the mRNA can be engineered to encode specific antigens from the tumor's mutations, stimulating a targeted immune response.

- **Viral Vector Vaccines** could be engineered to carry genetic material that's specifically suited to an individual's immune system, optimizing the body's defense mechanisms.

- **Protein Subunit Vaccines** can be tailored to deliver specific protein fragments that are most likely to induce the strongest immune response based on an individual's immune profile.

4. Personalized Vaccines for Cancer: A Promising Development

One of the most promising areas of personalized vaccine development is **cancer immunotherapy**. Cancer cells are often marked by mutations that are unique to each tumor. Personalized cancer vaccines seek to use these mutations as targets for the immune system, training it to recognize and destroy cancer cells while leaving healthy cells unharmed.

- **Neoantigen Vaccines**: The development of **neoantigen vaccines** is at the forefront of personalized cancer treatment. Neoantigens are abnormal proteins produced by tumor cells as a result of genetic mutations. By analyzing the tumor's genetic mutations, scientists can create a vaccine that teaches the immune system to recognize these unique antigens and specifically target the cancer cells.

- **Successes in Clinical Trials**: Some personalized cancer vaccines have already shown promise in early-phase clinical trials. For example, **BNT122**, an mRNA-based vaccine from BioNTech, is being tested as a personalized vaccine for melanoma. Other companies, like Moderna, are also working on personalized cancer vaccines, with promising early results for melanoma and other cancers.

5. Personalized Vaccines in Infectious Disease Prevention

While cancer is one of the most advanced fields for personalized vaccines, there are growing efforts to develop personalized vaccines for infectious diseases as well.

HIV Vaccines

HIV presents a significant challenge for vaccine development due to its ability to mutate rapidly and evade the immune system. A personalized HIV vaccine might use an individual's genetic makeup to predict how their immune system might respond to the virus and design a vaccine that targets specific regions of the virus. Personalized vaccines could also be used in combination with **gene editing** techniques like **CRISPR** to enhance the immune response and potentially offer long-term protection.

Influenza Vaccines

The flu virus also mutates frequently, and vaccines are often updated annually to match the circulating strain. Personalized influenza vaccines could use genetic profiling to predict which flu strain an individual is most likely to encounter, offering a more customized approach to flu prevention.

COVID-19 Vaccines

For COVID-19, personalized vaccines could be tailored to an individual's response to the virus, especially considering the variations in disease severity and immune response observed among different populations. Personalized vaccines could account for factors like **age**, **comorbidities**, and **genetic**

variations, ensuring a more precise immune response and better outcomes.

Challenges and Considerations for Personalized Vaccines

While the concept of personalized vaccines is promising, several challenges must be addressed before they can become mainstream:

1. **Cost and Accessibility**: Personalized vaccines are likely to be more expensive to produce and administer than traditional vaccines. The cost of genetic profiling, personalized vaccine development, and individualized treatment might limit access, particularly in low-income regions.

2. **Regulatory and Ethical Concerns**: The personalized vaccine approach will require new regulatory frameworks to ensure safety, efficacy, and equity in distribution. Ethical considerations, such as ensuring that genetic data is used responsibly and without discrimination, must also be addressed.

3. **Logistical Challenges**: Tailoring vaccines for each individual on a large scale poses significant logistical challenges in terms of production, distribution, and monitoring. Advances in **vaccine manufacturing** and **delivery systems** will be necessary to make personalized vaccines feasible at a global level.

The Future of Personalized Vaccines

The future of personalized vaccines holds tremendous potential, not just for improving vaccine effectiveness, but also for revolutionizing the way we think about disease prevention and treatment. By tailoring vaccines to the genetic makeup, health history, and environmental factors of each individual, we can create a more efficient and targeted approach to immunization. As research continues and technology evolves, personalized vaccines may become a key tool in eradicating infectious diseases, combating cancer, and improving overall global health.

In the coming decades, personalized vaccines could not only enhance our ability to prevent disease but also allow for more effective, long-lasting protection for each person based on their unique immune system. Ultimately, this precision medicine approach could be the key to ensuring that vaccines remain at the forefront of global health and disease prevention.

Preparing for Future Pandemics: The Role of Vaccines in Global Preparedness

The COVID-19 pandemic has highlighted the importance of rapid, effective responses to global health crises. Vaccines played a pivotal role in controlling the spread of the virus, preventing severe illness, and saving millions of lives. As we look to the future, preparing for potential pandemics will require a coordinated, global effort, with vaccines at the forefront of public health strategies. Understanding the role of vaccines in future pandemic preparedness is critical in building a resilient health infrastructure and ensuring swift, equitable access to immunization when the next outbreak occurs.

The Need for Pandemic Preparedness

Pandemics have been a recurring part of human history, from the Spanish Flu of 1918 to the more recent outbreaks of Ebola, Zika, and COVID-19. While the specific pathogens vary, the challenges they pose to global health systems are similar: the need for rapid detection, containment, treatment, and prevention. Vaccines have proven to be one of the most effective tools for preventing the spread of infectious diseases, but ensuring that vaccines can be developed and distributed quickly and equitably is a complex task that requires long-term planning and collaboration across countries, industries, and sectors.

The Role of Vaccines in Pandemic Preparedness

Vaccines are not only critical for controlling outbreaks once they occur but also serve as a cornerstone of pandemic preparedness. Here's how vaccines can contribute to managing and mitigating future pandemics:

1. Rapid Vaccine Development

One of the major lessons from the COVID-19 pandemic was the unprecedented speed at which vaccines were developed. The development of mRNA vaccines, in particular, showed that vaccines could be created and authorized for emergency use in a fraction of the time it would take for traditional vaccine platforms.

For future pandemics, preparing for rapid vaccine development is crucial. Investment in **vaccine platforms** that can be easily adapted to emerging infectious diseases, such as **mRNA vaccines**, **viral vector vaccines**, and **DNA vaccines**, will be essential. These platforms can be quickly modified to respond to new pathogens by encoding genetic material from the virus, allowing for faster development, clinical trials, and manufacturing processes.

- **mRNA Vaccine Technology**: As seen with COVID-19 vaccines, mRNA technology allows for a more streamlined approach to vaccine development. The ability to rapidly sequence a new pathogen's genome and design an mRNA vaccine based on that data means that vaccines can be produced within weeks, and large-scale manufacturing can follow soon after.

- **Universal Vaccines**: In addition to rapid development, scientists are working towards **universal vaccines** that could target a wide range of viruses within a family of pathogens. For instance, researchers are exploring **universal flu vaccines** and broader **coronavirus vaccines** that could provide protection against multiple strains and variants.

2. Stockpiling Vaccines and Vaccine Platforms

For future pandemics, it's critical to have an inventory of pre-produced vaccines or vaccine platforms ready to be deployed. Stockpiling vaccines, as well as the raw materials and production capabilities to make more when needed, is an essential part of pandemic preparedness. These stockpiles should be designed to cover a wide range of potential pathogens, including those that have yet to emerge.

Additionally, countries and international organizations can work together to establish **vaccine production hubs** that can scale up manufacturing when needed. This infrastructure, including the ability to rapidly produce large quantities of vaccines, would allow for faster distribution when an outbreak occurs.

3. Vaccine Distribution Systems

The ability to develop and produce vaccines quickly is important, but equally important is the ability to distribute them efficiently. Pandemic preparedness should include the establishment of **global vaccine distribution systems** that ensure equitable access to vaccines for all countries, especially low-income regions.

International organizations such as the **World Health Organization (WHO)**, **GAVI (Global Alliance for Vaccines and Immunization)**, and **UNICEF** have already demonstrated their capacity to support vaccine distribution, but there's room for improvement in terms of **logistics**, **transportation infrastructure**, and **supply chain resilience**. Pandemic vaccines need to be distributed swiftly, which means improving cold chain logistics, ensuring vaccine availability in hard-to-reach areas, and avoiding hoarding or unfair distribution practices.

- **COVAX Initiative**: The **COVAX initiative**, led by WHO and other partners, is an example of an international effort to ensure equitable vaccine access. Lessons from COVAX, particularly regarding distribution challenges and equitable access, can inform future pandemic preparedness strategies.

4. Vaccine Equity and Access

One of the most significant challenges during the COVID-19 pandemic was the disparity in vaccine access between high-income and low-income countries. Wealthier nations secured vaccine deals early, while low- and middle-income countries struggled to get sufficient doses, leading to widespread inequities in vaccination coverage.

To address this issue in future pandemics, global health systems must prioritize **vaccine equity**, ensuring that vaccines are distributed fairly, especially to countries and populations that are most vulnerable. This includes making vaccines affordable, providing technical support for vaccine delivery, and fostering international collaborations to ensure that all nations are prepared to respond to a pandemic.

- **Global Collaboration**: Governments, private companies, and non-governmental organizations must work together to ensure that vaccines are accessible to everyone, regardless of their country's economic status. This includes considering **tiered pricing**, **donations of vaccines**, and **technology transfer** to increase global manufacturing capacity.

5. Building Public Trust in Vaccination

Public trust in vaccines is critical for pandemic preparedness. During the COVID-19 pandemic, vaccine hesitancy became a major obstacle in many countries, even in the face of a highly effective vaccine. Misinformation, mistrust of government institutions, and fear of side effects all contributed to delays in vaccination campaigns.

In future pandemics, health authorities must build and maintain public trust by engaging in transparent, clear, and evidence-based communication. This includes providing accurate information about vaccine safety, efficacy, and the risks associated with not vaccinating. Public health campaigns should also address concerns and misconceptions about vaccination, especially during the early stages of a pandemic.

6. Vaccine Monitoring and Post-Vaccination Surveillance

After a vaccine is deployed, continuous monitoring and surveillance are essential to ensure its safety and effectiveness. This includes **vaccine safety monitoring** through systems like the **Vaccine Adverse Event Reporting System (VAERS)** and other surveillance networks to detect any potential adverse events and address them promptly.

Additionally, monitoring the effectiveness of vaccines in real-world conditions, especially in the context of new variants and evolving pathogens, is critical to understanding how vaccines perform over time. Adaptations to existing vaccines or the development of booster shots may be necessary to maintain immunity in the population.

7. Global Research and Innovation

Finally, a robust **global research** and **innovation ecosystem** will be vital in preparing for future pandemics. Funding for research into new vaccine technologies, including next-generation vaccines, **nanotechnology**, and **gene-based vaccines**, should be prioritized. International collaboration among scientists, governments, and private companies can help accelerate vaccine development, ensure the diversification of vaccine platforms, and increase preparedness for any emerging threats.

Conclusion

Vaccines will remain a central pillar of global health preparedness for future pandemics. Rapid development, equitable distribution, and the ability to adapt to new and emerging pathogens are essential components of pandemic readiness. By investing in innovative vaccine technologies, strengthening global collaborations, and ensuring vaccine equity, we can better prepare for the next global health crisis.

In the future, vaccines may not only be the key to preventing pandemics but also to ensuring that our global health systems can respond swiftly and effectively to the next outbreak, minimizing the impact on public health, economies, and society at large.

Ethical Considerations in Emerging Vaccine Technologies

As vaccine technology advances, ethical considerations become increasingly important in ensuring that new approaches are developed and deployed responsibly. Emerging vaccine technologies, such as mRNA vaccines, DNA vaccines, and personalized vaccines, offer the potential for more effective and rapid responses to infectious diseases, but they also present novel ethical challenges. These challenges include concerns about safety, equity, informed consent, privacy, and the potential unintended consequences of new technologies.

1. Safety and Long-Term Effects

One of the primary ethical concerns with emerging vaccine technologies is ensuring their safety and addressing the uncertainty regarding their long-term effects. While technologies like mRNA and DNA vaccines have shown promise in clinical trials, they are still relatively new compared to traditional vaccine platforms. This raises questions about their long-term impact on human health.

- **Ethical Challenge**: Should these vaccines be widely distributed before their long-term safety profiles are fully understood?

- **Considerations**: Researchers and regulators must ensure that adequate clinical trials are conducted to assess the long-term safety of new vaccine platforms. Ethical guidelines should emphasize transparent communication with the public regarding the risks and benefits of new technologies. It is critical to maintain rigorous monitoring systems post-market, such as the **Vaccine Adverse Event Reporting System (VAERS)**, to detect and address any adverse events that may arise.

2. Informed Consent and Public Trust

As emerging vaccine technologies are developed, ensuring informed consent becomes a significant ethical concern. The concept of informed consent means that individuals must be given clear, accurate information about the risks, benefits, and potential unknowns associated with the vaccine. In the case of novel technologies, there may be limited understanding of long-term effects, which complicates the informed consent process.

- **Ethical Challenge**: How can health authorities ensure that individuals are adequately informed about the new vaccine technologies, especially when there may be gaps in public understanding or fear of unknown risks?

- **Considerations**: Clear communication is essential in fostering trust in vaccine technologies. Health officials should be transparent about what is known, what is uncertain, and how risks are being monitored. Informed consent forms should be accessible, comprehensible, and in languages or formats that are easily understood by diverse populations.

3. Equity in Access to New Vaccine Technologies

Emerging vaccine technologies often come with high research and development costs, which can result in limited access to vaccines, particularly in low- and middle-income countries. This raises ethical concerns regarding the equitable distribution of vaccines.

- **Ethical Challenge**: How can we ensure that new vaccine technologies are accessible to all populations, particularly vulnerable and marginalized groups?

- **Considerations**: Global collaborations, such as the **COVAX initiative**, can help ensure that vaccines are distributed equitably worldwide. Vaccine manufacturers and governments should work together to develop strategies for ensuring that emerging vaccines are affordable, available, and accessible in underserved regions. Public health policies should include measures to prioritize access to vaccines for high-risk populations, regardless of socioeconomic status or geographic location.

4. Privacy and Genetic Information

With the development of DNA and mRNA vaccines, there is increasing concern about the collection and use of genetic data. For example, some vaccine technologies involve analyzing a person's genetic makeup to personalize the vaccine or to assess their risk of side effects.

- **Ethical Challenge**: How can we ensure that genetic data used in vaccine development or personalized vaccines is protected and not misused?

- **Considerations**: Strict privacy protections must be in place to safeguard personal genetic information. Individuals should be made aware of how their genetic data will be used, stored, and shared. Consent protocols should be transparent, and genetic data should only be used for its intended purpose. Additionally, there should be regulations in place to prevent the misuse of genetic information, such as for genetic discrimination in insurance or employment.

5. The Right to Refuse Emerging Vaccines

Emerging vaccines often spark debates about autonomy and individual rights, especially when new technologies are introduced rapidly. Some individuals may question the necessity of using novel vaccine technologies or may refuse to be vaccinated due to concerns over safety or the lack of long-term data.

- **Ethical Challenge**: What is the balance between individual autonomy and the collective responsibility of vaccination for public health?

- **Considerations**: It is essential to respect individual rights while also considering the broader public health benefits of vaccination. Public health campaigns should aim to educate and inform the public about the benefits of vaccines, addressing concerns and misconceptions. At the same time, governments may need to navigate the delicate balance between respecting personal autonomy and ensuring herd immunity to protect vulnerable populations.

6. Dual-Use Technology and Military Applications

Some emerging vaccine technologies, especially those based on genetic modifications or biotechnologies, have the potential for dual-use — meaning they could be used for both beneficial and harmful purposes. There are concerns that technologies originally developed for public health purposes could be repurposed for military or bioweapons research.

- **Ethical Challenge**: How can we ensure that vaccine technologies are used only for their intended public health benefits and not for harmful or malicious purposes?

- **Considerations**: Strict oversight and international agreements should regulate the use of emerging vaccine technologies, ensuring that they are developed, distributed, and used ethically. This includes monitoring for potential misuse and ensuring that the technology is not diverted for harmful purposes.

7. The Risk of Unintended Consequences

Novel vaccine platforms, such as mRNA vaccines, operate in new ways, and their full effects on the body are not yet entirely known. While initial data suggests their safety and efficacy, unforeseen side effects or long-term health consequences may arise as these vaccines are used on a larger scale.

- **Ethical Challenge**: How can we mitigate the risks of unintended consequences when deploying emerging vaccine technologies, particularly when there may be unknowns about their long-term effects?

- **Considerations**: Ongoing research, surveillance, and the use of post-market monitoring systems will be essential to detecting and addressing unintended consequences. Ethical frameworks should emphasize the need for continuous monitoring and the ability to respond quickly to any new findings related to vaccine safety. In cases of severe adverse events, there should be transparent and accountable procedures for compensation and support for affected individuals.

8. The Potential for 'Vaccine Passports' and Discrimination

As the world moves toward greater vaccination coverage, some nations and organizations are considering the use of "vaccine passports" or digital certificates to verify that individuals have been vaccinated against certain diseases. While these passports could help facilitate safe travel and participation in society, they also raise concerns about privacy, surveillance, and discrimination.

- **Ethical Challenge**: How can we balance the benefits of vaccination verification systems with the protection of individual rights and privacy?

- **Considerations**: Governments and organizations should establish clear guidelines about how vaccine passports are implemented, ensuring that they do not discriminate against those who are unable or unwilling to be vaccinated for legitimate reasons. Policies should also consider how to protect individuals' privacy and personal data, ensuring that the information collected is not misused or shared without consent.

Conclusion

Emerging vaccine technologies have the potential to revolutionize global health, but they also introduce complex ethical dilemmas that must be carefully addressed. Ensuring safety, equity, privacy, and public trust while respecting individual autonomy and rights will be key to the successful deployment of these technologies. Policymakers, researchers, and health authorities must work together to navigate these ethical challenges, ensuring that the benefits of emerging vaccines are realized without compromising ethical standards or public confidence.

Chapter 10: Navigating the Vaccine Debate as a Parent or Concerned Citizen

How to Make Informed Decisions About Vaccines

Making informed decisions about vaccines is crucial for ensuring the health of yourself, your family, and your community. With so much information—both accurate and misleading—available online, navigating the vaccine debate can feel overwhelming. This guide will help you make thoughtful, evidence-based decisions about vaccination by offering key strategies to evaluate information and consider both scientific facts and your personal circumstances.

1. Start with Reliable, Credible Sources

The first step in making an informed decision is to seek information from trustworthy and evidence-based sources. Here are some organizations and resources you can rely on for accurate information:

- **Health Authorities**: Reputable organizations like the **Centers for Disease Control and Prevention (CDC)**, the **World Health Organization (WHO)**, and the **American Academy of Pediatrics (AAP)** provide clear, reliable guidelines and information about vaccines.

- **Your Healthcare Provider**: Doctors and pediatricians are well-equipped to answer your questions about vaccines and can offer personalized advice based on your family's medical history. They can address concerns, explain the benefits and risks, and clarify any misconceptions.

- **Peer-Reviewed Research**: Look for studies published in respected medical journals that have been through rigorous peer review. These studies often provide the most accurate and up-to-date information on vaccine safety and effectiveness.

2. Understand How Vaccines Work

Before making a decision about vaccines, it's important to understand how they work and why they are necessary. Vaccines help the immune system recognize and fight harmful pathogens by introducing small, harmless pieces of the pathogen (like proteins or genetic material). This process stimulates the body to produce antibodies that protect against future infections.

- **Vaccine Safety**: Vaccines undergo extensive clinical trials and regulatory scrutiny before being approved for use. They are safe for the vast majority of individuals, with side effects that are typically mild and temporary.

- **Vaccine Efficacy**: Vaccines have been proven to significantly reduce the incidence of diseases. For example, vaccines have helped eliminate diseases like smallpox and have drastically reduced the incidence of polio, measles, and other deadly illnesses.

3. Consider the Risks of Vaccination

While vaccines are safe, no medical intervention is without some level of risk. However, serious adverse events from vaccines are extremely rare. Most people experience only mild side effects, such as soreness at the injection site or a slight fever. These side effects usually resolve on their own within a few days.

If you have concerns about vaccines and their potential risks, it's important to discuss them with a healthcare provider who can provide evidence-based answers tailored to your situation.

4. Evaluate the Risks of Not Vaccinating

The decision not to vaccinate can have serious consequences for both individual and public health. Unvaccinated individuals are at a higher risk of contracting and spreading diseases, which can lead to serious illness or death. Additionally, some individuals (such as infants, the elderly, and people with compromised immune systems) cannot be vaccinated or may be more vulnerable to diseases.

- **Herd Immunity**: By vaccinating yourself and your family, you contribute to herd immunity, which protects vulnerable individuals who cannot receive vaccines or those who may have weakened immune systems.

5. Question Misinformation and Myths

Misinformation about vaccines is widespread, especially on social media platforms, where claims about vaccines causing various health issues (e.g., autism) are often propagated without scientific evidence. To avoid falling victim to myths, consider these tips:

- **Seek Evidence-Based Information**: Look for data from credible sources and studies, not anecdotes or unverified claims. Vaccines are rigorously tested for safety, and their benefits have been proven through decades of research.

- **Check the Source**: Be wary of information from non-experts, as misinformation can easily spread in non-peer-reviewed spaces. Always verify claims with trusted organizations like the CDC or WHO.

- **Understand the Science**: If you come across a claim that seems questionable, do some research to understand how vaccines work and how scientific studies evaluate their safety and effectiveness.

6. Understand the Role of Vaccines in Public Health

Vaccines are not just about protecting individuals—they are a critical part of public health strategies to prevent outbreaks and control the spread of disease. The widespread adoption of vaccines has dramatically reduced the incidence of many infectious diseases that once caused widespread suffering and death.

- **Global Impact**: Vaccines have played a key role in eradicating smallpox and nearly eradicating polio, and they continue to save millions of lives each year worldwide.

- **Preventing Future Outbreaks**: Vaccination is one of the most effective ways to prevent the spread of infectious diseases. By vaccinating, we protect not only ourselves but also our communities, especially those who are most vulnerable.

7. Engage with Healthcare Providers

If you are unsure about the decision to vaccinate, one of the best steps you can take is to engage in a conversation with a trusted healthcare provider. They can address any specific concerns you may have, help you understand the benefits and risks in the context of your health history, and offer advice tailored to your family's needs.

- **Prepare Questions**: Before meeting with a healthcare provider, it can be helpful to write down any questions or concerns you may have. Some common questions might include:

  - Are there any specific risks for my child based on their medical history?

  - How do the benefits of vaccination outweigh the risks?

  - How do vaccines contribute to herd immunity?

8. Be Open to New Information

The field of medicine, including vaccine science, is constantly evolving. Stay informed by regularly checking trusted sources for updates on new vaccines, recommendations, or scientific findings. Vaccination schedules and guidelines may change as new vaccines are developed or as research provides new insights into vaccine safety and efficacy.

9. Take into Account Your Family's Health Needs

Each person's health situation is unique, and it's important to consider how vaccination fits into your or your family's overall health strategy. For example, individuals with compromised immune systems or certain allergies may need special considerations or alternatives for certain vaccines. Work closely with healthcare professionals to understand any adjustments that may be necessary for your personal circumstances.

Conclusion: Empower Yourself with Knowledge

Making an informed decision about vaccines is about understanding the science, considering the risks and benefits, and seeking trustworthy information. Vaccines are one of the most effective ways to protect yourself, your family, and your community from serious diseases. By approaching the vaccine debate with an open mind and a commitment to evidence-based decision-making, you can make choices that support not just your health, but the health of those around you.

In the end, the decision to vaccinate should be based on scientific facts, expert advice, and careful consideration of how it impacts both individual and public health.

Trusting Science: Separating Fact from Fiction

In an age where information is abundant and easily accessible, it can be difficult to distinguish between fact and fiction, especially when it comes to topics as important as vaccines. Misinformation and conspiracy theories can spread quickly, especially on social media, leading to confusion, fear, and distrust. It's more important than ever to understand how science works and how to separate reliable, evidence-based facts from myths and misconceptions.

Here are key strategies for trusting science and making informed decisions, particularly about vaccines:

1. Understanding the Scientific Method

Science is a systematic way of gathering knowledge and testing ideas. The scientific method involves forming a hypothesis, conducting experiments, analyzing data, and drawing conclusions based on evidence. The goal is to understand the world around us through repeatable, observable, and measurable results.

- **Hypothesis**: A proposed explanation based on observations.

- **Experimentation**: Controlled tests that examine whether the hypothesis holds true.

- **Data Analysis**: Interpreting the results of experiments to understand their meaning.

- **Peer Review**: Other scientists evaluate the methods, results, and conclusions of a study to ensure its validity.

In the context of vaccines, the scientific method is applied through years of rigorous research, clinical trials, and ongoing monitoring to assess their safety and effectiveness.

2. Evaluating Sources of Information

In today's digital age, not all information is created equal. It's essential to evaluate the sources of information you encounter, especially when it comes to topics like vaccine safety and efficacy. Here's how to identify trustworthy sources:

- **Reputable Organizations**: Seek information from well-established, scientifically credible organizations, such as the **Centers for Disease Control and Prevention (CDC)**, the **World Health Organization (WHO)**, and other public health agencies. These institutions base their guidelines on the latest scientific research.

- **Peer-Reviewed Journals**: Scientific studies published in peer-reviewed journals, such as **The Lancet** or the **New England Journal of Medicine**, are subject to review by experts in the field. This process helps ensure that the research is valid and reliable.

- **Scientific Experts**: Look to medical professionals, epidemiologists, and scientists who have dedicated their careers to studying infectious diseases, immunology, and vaccine safety. Their work is grounded in evidence and rigorous research.

- **Beware of Unverified Claims**: Misinformation often originates from unverified or unqualified sources. Websites, blogs, and social media posts that do not provide evidence or rely on personal stories rather than scientific data should be viewed with caution.

3. The Importance of Peer Review

One of the most important elements of scientific research is **peer review**. Peer review is a process in which experts in the field examine a study's methodology, data, and conclusions before it is published. This ensures that the research is credible and that any potential errors or biases are addressed.

In the case of vaccine studies, peer-reviewed research helps confirm that vaccines are both safe and effective. While no study is perfect, the peer review process helps ensure that studies meet high standards of scientific integrity.

4. Understanding the Evidence Behind Vaccines

The effectiveness and safety of vaccines are not based on anecdotes or isolated stories, but on large bodies of evidence collected over time. Consider the following:

- **Clinical Trials**: Before any vaccine is approved, it undergoes extensive clinical trials involving tens of thousands of participants. These trials test for safety, effectiveness, and potential side effects across various populations.

- **Real-World Data**: Once a vaccine is approved, its safety and effectiveness are continuously monitored through systems like the **Vaccine Adverse Event Reporting System (VAERS)** and post-market surveillance. This allows experts to track any long-term effects or rare side effects.

- **Epidemiological Studies**: Large-scale population studies examine how vaccines impact disease rates over time. These studies have shown that vaccines prevent millions of deaths and hospitalizations every year by controlling infectious diseases.

5. The Role of Consensus in Science

In science, **consensus** is reached when the majority of experts agree on a particular finding based on available evidence. In the case of vaccines, a strong consensus exists among medical and scientific communities that vaccines are safe and effective in preventing serious diseases.

This consensus is formed through years of rigorous research, studies, and real-world evidence. For instance, multiple large-scale studies have shown that vaccines do not cause autism, debunking one of the most persistent myths. The overwhelming scientific consensus is that vaccines have saved millions of lives and have contributed to the decline of deadly diseases.

6. The Impact of Misinformation on Public Health

Misinformation, especially about vaccines, can have serious consequences for public health. False claims, such as vaccines causing autism or being unsafe, can lead to vaccine hesitancy and outbreaks of preventable diseases. It's important to recognize how misinformation spreads and to be critical of sources that promote unverified or sensational claims.

- **Fear and Uncertainty**: Misleading information often preys on people's fears and uncertainties, presenting one-sided arguments without context or evidence. To counter this, focus on reliable scientific sources and seek answers from experts who can clarify complex issues with facts and evidence.

- **Vaccine Hesitancy**: One of the key reasons for vaccine hesitancy is misinformation. Studies show that people who are uncertain about vaccines often express concerns after being exposed to false or misleading information. Addressing misinformation through education and open dialogue can help build trust in vaccines.

7. How to Engage with the Science of Vaccines

To trust science, it's important to engage with the facts and be open to learning. Here's how you can build your understanding and trust in vaccines:

- **Ask Questions**: If you're unsure about vaccines or the information you've come across, ask healthcare professionals or scientists for clarification. They can provide clear, evidence-based explanations that are rooted in scientific research.

- **Stay Informed**: Follow reputable sources and keep up with the latest research. Vaccines, like all medical treatments, are continuously monitored and studied, and new insights are shared regularly.

- **Challenge Misinformation**: If you encounter false claims about vaccines, challenge them by pointing to credible, scientifically-backed information. It's important to share facts that can help dispel myths and encourage informed decision-making.

8. Trusting Science in the Face of Uncertainty

It's natural to feel uncertain when faced with new information or complex topics like vaccines. However, trusting science doesn't mean having all the answers right away—it means being open to learning and adjusting your views based on credible, evidence-based information. The scientific community continuously tests hypotheses, reviews data, and adapts to new findings, ensuring that conclusions are based on the best available evidence.

Conclusion: The Importance of Trusting Science

The vaccine debate can be complicated, but by trusting science and relying on credible sources, you can make informed decisions that protect your health and the health of your community. Vaccines are a vital tool in preventing disease, and the scientific evidence supporting their safety and effectiveness is robust and undeniable. By understanding how science works, critically evaluating sources of information, and separating fact from fiction, you can navigate the complex landscape of vaccine information with confidence and clarity.

Talking to Others About Vaccines: What to Say and How to Listen

Discussing vaccines, especially with someone who may be hesitant or misinformed, can be challenging. However, these conversations are essential for promoting understanding and trust in vaccines. By approaching these discussions with empathy, respect, and accurate information, you can play a crucial role in addressing concerns and encouraging informed decisions. Here are some strategies for engaging in productive conversations about vaccines.

1. Approach the Conversation with Empathy

The first step in any conversation about vaccines is to approach it with empathy and understanding. People's views on vaccines may be influenced by personal experiences, cultural beliefs, or exposure to misinformation. It's important to recognize that vaccine hesitancy is often driven by fear, uncertainty, or misinformation, rather than malice.

- **Acknowledge their concerns**: Begin by acknowledging that their concerns or questions are valid. Showing empathy helps create an open and respectful space for dialogue.

- **Listen actively**: Ask questions to understand where they are coming from and listen carefully to their points of view. Active listening builds trust and opens the door for constructive discussion.

Example: "I understand that you're worried about the safety of vaccines. Can you tell me more about what you've heard or what concerns you?"

2. Use Facts, Not Confrontation

While it may be tempting to challenge someone's views directly or present a barrage of facts, such an approach can lead to defensiveness and make the person less open to hearing the information. Instead, focus on calmly presenting evidence and addressing their specific concerns.

- **Stick to the science**: Present evidence-based information from credible sources like the CDC, WHO, or trusted medical professionals. Explain how vaccines are rigorously tested for safety and effectiveness before they are approved for use.

- **Provide context**: Sometimes people misunderstand the numbers or statistics they hear. When discussing vaccine safety, for example, be sure to explain how rare adverse events are compared to the benefits of preventing serious diseases.

Example: "The CDC monitors vaccine safety continuously, and the risk of a serious side effect is extremely low—far lower than the risk of getting the diseases that vaccines prevent."

3. Be Patient and Avoid Judging

Changing someone's mind about vaccines takes time, and pushing too hard or making them feel judged can backfire. It's important to remain patient and recognize that the goal is to foster a dialogue, not to win an argument.

- **Be patient**: Some people need time to process information and may not immediately change their stance. Offer to continue the conversation and provide them with resources they can explore at their own pace.

- **Avoid using judgmental language**: Instead of labeling someone as "anti-vaccine" or "misinformed," focus on the shared goal of protecting health. Acknowledge that everyone wants what's best for their family and community.

Example: "I totally understand why you might be feeling uncertain about vaccines—it's a big decision. I've read a lot about this myself, and I'd love to share some of the information that helped me feel more comfortable."

4. Provide Reliable Resources

In conversations about vaccines, providing access to credible, reliable resources can help combat misinformation. Offer materials from trusted medical organizations and encourage the person to read or explore them.

- **Direct them to authoritative sources**: Websites like the CDC, WHO, and local public health organizations provide clear, fact-based information about vaccine safety, effectiveness, and potential side effects.

- **Suggest peer-reviewed articles or studies**: If the person is open to more detailed information, provide them with scientific studies or articles that demonstrate the safety and benefits of vaccines.

Example: "Here's a great article from the CDC that talks about how vaccines are tested for safety and what's involved in making sure they're effective."

5. Share Personal Stories and Testimonials

Personal stories can be powerful in illustrating the benefits of vaccines. If you've had positive experiences with vaccines or know someone whose life was protected by immunization, sharing these stories can help make the abstract concept of vaccination more relatable.

- **Share your own experience**: Talk about how getting vaccinated has protected you or your family from preventable diseases.

- **Use stories of people you know**: Personal testimonials from people who have experienced the benefits of vaccination, or who have had their lives affected by vaccine-preventable diseases, can be very compelling.

Example: "I know a family whose child nearly contracted a preventable disease. Fortunately, they were vaccinated, and it made all the difference in protecting them."

6. Discuss the Broader Social Benefits of Vaccination

Beyond personal protection, vaccines have significant societal benefits. One of the most important roles of vaccines is contributing to **herd immunity**, which helps protect those who cannot be vaccinated due to medical reasons, such as infants or people with compromised immune systems.

- **Explain herd immunity**: Help the person understand how vaccination protects not only the individual but also vulnerable members of the community.

- **Highlight the importance of collective responsibility**: Vaccines are a collective effort to ensure that infectious diseases do not spread and affect the most vulnerable members of society.

Example: "By getting vaccinated, you're not just protecting yourself, but also people who can't get vaccinated, like babies or people with weakened immune systems."

7. Address Specific Concerns with Evidence

People may have specific concerns about vaccines, such as their safety, ingredients, or potential side effects. Address these concerns directly, using scientific evidence to provide clear, well-researched answers.

- **Safety and side effects**: Explain that vaccines are thoroughly tested for safety and are monitored for adverse events once they're approved. Make it clear that side effects are rare and usually mild.

- **Ingredients**: Clarify any misconceptions about vaccine ingredients. Many people are concerned about substances like mercury or aluminum, but vaccines contain only trace amounts of these substances, and they are used safely in much larger quantities in other contexts (e.g., in everyday foods).

Example: "I understand that you're concerned about the ingredients in vaccines. The amount of mercury in vaccines, for example, is so tiny that it's far less than the amount we encounter in things like fish, which many of us eat regularly."

8. Respect Autonomy While Offering Information

It's essential to respect the autonomy of the person you're speaking with. People need to make their own decisions, and trying to force a viewpoint on someone can be counterproductive. Instead, focus on providing clear, factual information and support them in making the decision that feels right for them.

- **Respect their choice**: If they are not ready to get vaccinated, acknowledge their decision and offer information that might help them reconsider in the future. Keep the door open for ongoing conversations.

Example: "I completely understand if you're not ready to make a decision right now. Just know that I'm here to talk and share information whenever you're ready."

9. Know When to End the Conversation

Sometimes, despite your best efforts, the conversation may not be productive. It's important to recognize when the person is not receptive to new information. Rather than forcing the discussion, offer resources for further reading and let them know that you're available to talk in the future.

- **Leave the door open**: Let them know that they can come back to you with any questions or if they want to discuss things further.

Example: "I know this is a lot to think about, but if you ever have more questions, feel free to reach out to me. I'd be happy to share more information."

Conclusion: Creating Constructive Conversations About Vaccines

Talking about vaccines with others can be a rewarding opportunity to share knowledge and promote health, but it requires a thoughtful approach. By approaching the conversation with empathy, listening actively, providing reliable information, and respecting the other person's perspective, you can help create a space for constructive dialogue. Even if opinions don't change immediately, these conversations contribute to building understanding, which can lead to better decisions for individuals and communities in the long run.

Conclusion

Vaccination is one of the most effective tools in preventing disease and protecting public health. However, the complexities of vaccine development, the challenges of addressing vaccine hesitancy, and the evolving nature of infectious diseases present significant hurdles in ensuring widespread immunization. Throughout this book, we have explored the science behind vaccines, the historical success of vaccination campaigns, the ethical and societal debates surrounding mandates, and the global efforts to ensure equitable access to vaccines.

Informed decision-making is the cornerstone of addressing vaccine hesitancy and misinformation. As we have seen, vaccines are not only a matter of individual health but also a collective responsibility. Herd immunity, the global eradication of diseases like smallpox and polio, and the continued fight against emerging infectious threats underscore the importance of vaccination.

It is essential to trust in scientific research, seek out credible sources of information, and remain open to conversations about the benefits and risks of vaccines. By fostering open dialogue, supporting vaccine access in underserved regions, and embracing emerging vaccine technologies, we can continue to protect ourselves, our communities, and future generations from preventable diseases.

Ultimately, the future of vaccination relies on the shared commitment of individuals, healthcare providers, public health organizations, and governments to ensure that science, equity, and public health priorities guide our path forward. Vaccines have already transformed global health, and with continued innovation, education, and collaboration, we can build a healthier, more resilient world for all.

Made in the USA
Monee, IL
24 November 2024

71071314R00144